PALEO

Publications International, Ltd.

Louis Weber, CEO
Publications International, Ltd.
7373 North Cicero Avenue
Lincolnwood, IL 60712

Pictured on the front cover *(clockwise from top):* Beef Tenderloin with High Spice Rub *(page 48),* Avocado Salsa *(page 178),* Spicy Crabmeat Frittata *(page 14)* and Balsamic Butternut Squash *(page 174).*

Pictured on the back cover *(clockwise from left):* Coconut Shrimp with Pear Chutney *(page 158),* Sage-Roasted Pork with Rutabaga *(page 104)* and Tangy Red Cabbage with Apples and Bacon *(page 180).*

Contributing Writer: Marilyn Pocius

ISBN: 978-1-4508-8460-0

Library of Congress Control Number: 2014933999

Manufactured in China.

8 7 6 5 4 3 2 1

Microwave Cooking: Microwave ovens vary in wattage. Use the cooking times as guidelines and check for doneness before adding more time.

Publications International, Ltd.

TABLE OF CONTENTS

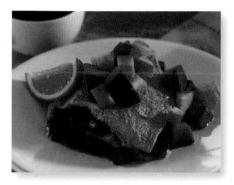

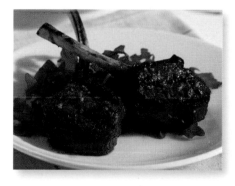

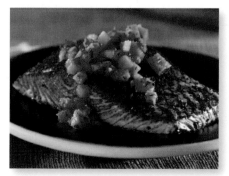

4   The Paleo Principles

10   Eggs

18   Poultry

48   Beef

78   Pork

108   Lamb

122   Fish

150   Shellfish

166   Sides & Snacks

187   Index

A NEW DIET THAT'S 100,000 YEARS OLD: PALEO

Humans were hunter-gatherers for tens of thousands of years. They ate the wild plants they could find and the meat they could kill. Why should we care what they ate? One reason is that after all these centuries, our DNA is still virtually identical to theirs.

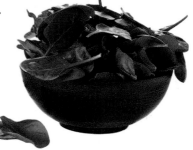

The most profound and recent change in the way humans live and eat resulted from the invention of agriculture, which began less than 10,000 years ago—a mere drop in the bucket in evolutionary history. Agriculture allowed us to go from a diet of lean meat and lots of different kinds of fruits and vegetables to one based primarily on grains and starchy crops.

There is quite a lot of anthropological evidence that this change was not healthy for Homo sapiens. Studies of early agricultural societies indicate that they had shorter life spans, more malnutrition and were shorter in stature than their Paleolithic forebears. Agriculture allowed us to stay in one place, to feed more people and to develop culture. Nobody wants to go back to the Stone Age. But since our genetic make-up hasn't changed, maybe, just maybe, the modern high-carb, low-fat diet isn't the ideal for us.

Paleo Made Simple

1. Eat whole foods, not processed

2. Don't eat grains (especially wheat, but also corn, rice, oats, barley)

3. Eliminate dairy products

4. Avoid legumes (beans, peanuts)

5. Enjoy lots of vegetables and plenty of protein

BUT I'M NOT A CAVEMAN!

Our lives are (thank heavens!) very different, but our digestive systems may not be. Obviously we can't literally eat what Paleo man did. Nobody wants to dine on bison brain with a side of bitter greens. What the Paleo diet proposes is that we learn from what worked and find modern healthy equivalents. It's not complicated. It's an invitation to change your diet from mostly processed, refined carbohydrates to whole foods, protein, carbohydrates from fruits and vegetables, and good fats.

THE PALEO PANTRY

WHAT'S IN:

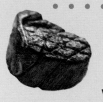

Meats: Bacon, Beef, Buffalo, Lamb, Pork, Veal, Venison

Poultry: Chicken, Duck, Quail, Turkey

Eggs (preferably organic and pasture-raised)

Seafood: Catfish, Clams, Halibut, Herring, Lobster, Mahimahi, Mussels, Salmon, Sardines, Scallops, Shrimp, Trout, Tuna

Fats and Oils: Butter (grass-fed), Coconut oil, Nut oils, Olive oil, Palm oil

Vegetables: Artichokes, Arugula, Asparagus, Broccoli, Brussels sprouts, Cabbage, Carrots, Cauliflower, Celery, Chard, Cucumbers, Eggplant, Fennel, Garlic, Green beans, Kale, Kohlrabi, Leeks, Lettuce, Mushrooms, Onions, Parsnips, Peppers, Radishes, Rutabagas, Spinach, Squash, Sweet potatoes, Tomatoes

Fruits: Apricots, Avocados, Bananas, Blackberries, Blueberries, Cherries, Coconut, Cranberries, Figs, Grapefruit, Grapes, Kiwis, Lemons, Limes, Mangoes, Melons, Nectarines, Oranges, Papayas, Peaches, Pears, Pineapples, Plums, Pomegranates, Raspberries, Rhubarb, Strawberries, Tangerines, Watermelon

Nuts and Seeds: Almonds, Brazil nuts, Hazelnuts, Macadamia nuts, Pecans, Pine nuts, Pistachios, Pumpkin seeds, Sesame seeds, Sunflower seeds, Walnuts

Flavorings: Capers, Coconut aminos, Fresh and dried herbs, Ginger, Lemon and lime juice, Mustard, Vanilla, Vinegars (balsamic, cider, wine), Whole and ground spices

WHAT'S OUT:

Processed Foods

Grains: Barley, Corn, Oats, Millet, Quinoa, Rice, Rye, Wheat and products containing them or containing gluten

Prepared/Packaged Carbs: Bagels, Baked goods, Biscuits, Breads, Breakfast and snack bars, Cereal, Chips, Cookies, Crackers, Muffins, Pasta, Pretzels, Scones, Tacos

Dairy: Cheese, Ice cream, Milk, Yogurt (see page 9 for exceptions)

Legumes: Beans, Chickpeas, Soybeans and soy products, Peanuts

Processed Vegetable Oils: Canola oil, Corn oil, Margarine and "buttery" spreads, Peanut oil, Shortening, Vegetable oil

Sugar and Artificial Sweeteners: Brown, cane and powdered sugar, Corn syrup, Dextrose, Sucrose or products containing them

SO WHAT'S FOR DINNER (AND BREAKFAST AND LUNCH)?

A glance at the Paleo pantry and the many wonderful recipes in this book should give you some good ideas. If you've been eating a typical modern diet of fast food, pasta, bread and sweets, Paleo does take adjustments. You'll spend more time shopping and cooking and being mindful of what you eat—and that's a good thing.

What's the difference between Paleo, low carb and gluten-free?

There are similarities, but the basic premise of the Paleo diet is to eat only whole, unprocessed foods. Most low-carb regimens are designed for quick weight loss and require limiting some fruits and vegetables. Gluten-free diets are for those with celiac disease or other sensitivities to the protein in wheat.

EAT ENOUGH PROTEIN.

Meat (especially red meat), poultry and eggs have been maligned for years since they contain cholesterol and saturated fat. They do, but as you have probably noticed, nutritional guidelines change over time. Once egg yolks were forbidden because they raised cholesterol. Then we learned that there are many kinds of cholesterol that your body needs and what we eat may not increase the amount in our bloodstreams. Will eating red meat put you in immediate danger of a heart attack? Not so fast. It depends on what else you're eating, what kind of meat it is and dozens of other factors.

To stick to the Paleo plan you need the simplest, highest quality protein you can find and afford. The best choices are pasture-raised, grass-fed meat and eggs. This is easy to understand if you remember that animals raised on a feedlot and fattened on corn are not remotely like the lean, free-range animals our ancestors consumed.

Pasture-raised meat contains a larger proportion of beneficial omega-3 fatty acids, the same helpful nutrient that is in fish oil and is sadly lacking in the modern diet. When choosing supermarket meat, go for leaner cuts. Most importantly, avoid any processed product that has been "enhanced," marinated or pre-seasoned. Look for eggs from chickens that are fed a diet that increases the content of omega-3s where pasture-raised is hard to find or too expensive.

CHOOSE HIGH QUALITY SEAFOOD.

As with meat, the closer seafood is to its natural state, the better. If you can't go fishing yourself, look for wild-caught fish and purchase from a reputable source that has a high turnover. Pay attention to country of origin when purchasing shrimp. The best choice is U.S. farmed. Imported products can be raised in polluted waters.

ENJOY LOTS OF VEGETABLES AT BREAKFAST, LUNCH AND DINNER.

No need to count calories or carbs when it comes to vegetables. It's practically impossible to overeat broccoli or salad greens. Most Paleo diets eliminate potatoes, but sweet potatoes are permitted. (They're botanically unrelated to white potatoes.)

Take this opportunity to try new and different vegetables. How about a frittata with fresh spinach (page 12) for breakfast? Dress up your lunchtime salad with artichoke hearts. Make crunchy chips from beets or kale for a snack. Roast parsnips, carrots and rutabaga drizzled with olive oil as a side dish. Add fennel, sweet peppers and onions to roast chicken.

SATISFY YOUR SWEET TOOTH WITH FRUIT.

Fruit will always taste best and be most nutritious when it is in season. Visit local farmers' markets for great selections. Shopping there may be as close as we can get to hunting and gathering! Remember that fruits contain fructose, which is sugar, and some can be high in carbs. If you're not losing weight and you wish to, try cutting back a little. Be careful of concentrated carbs and sugars in dried fruits and check ingredient lists for hidden sugars.

CHOOSE THE RIGHT KINDS OF FATS.

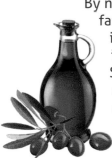

By now you've probably accepted that it's not fat that makes us fat. Our fat storage system is dependent on insulin, and insulin levels increase in response to carbohydrates. Still, the kind of fat we eat does matter. The saturated fat found in red meat used to be considered unhealthy, but that's certainly what Paleo man ate. There were no manufactured vegetable oils.

Did we improve on nature by switching from saturated fat to polyunsaturated vegetable oils? Probably not. What we did do was drastically change the ratio of omega-3 fatty acids to omega-6 fatty acids in our diets. Omega-3s come from grass-fed meats and wild-caught fish. Vegetable oils, including corn, canola and soy, are the primary source of excess omega-6 fatty acids today. This lack of balance is the reason for the increasing interest in fish oil capsules and flaxseed, which are high in omega-3s.

What this means is that you should avoid processed polyunsaturated oils and, of course, trans fats. Instead use olive oil, coconut oil or butter from pasture-raised cows. Wherever possible, eat grass-fed meats instead of corn-fed factory-farmed animals.

Coconut Aminos

Made from the sap of the coconut palm, this bottled product can be a replacement for soy sauce. In addition to being made from soy beans, traditional soy sauce also has added wheat, so it contains gluten. Coconut aminos can be used in stir-fries, dressings and wherever you would use soy sauce.

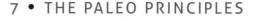

KEEP THINGS INTERESTING WITH NUTS, SEEDS, HERBS AND SPICES.

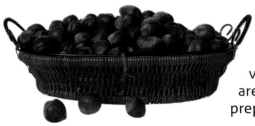

Making meals and snacks pleasurable doesn't have to mean spending more money or time. Almond or macadamia butter can easily replace peanut butter with your sliced apples. Herbs and spices can add endless variation to the simplest preparations. Herbs and spices are all paleo, but watch ingredient lists if you're purchasing prepared blends. They often contain sugar in some form.

GIVING UP GRAIN

How can wheat, corn, soy, oats, rice and rye be bad for us? They are all domesticated forms of wild grasses that have been managed and "improved" by agriculture for 5,000 years. Remember, that's a short time in terms of human evolution. Wheat, barley and rye contain a protein called gluten. Other grains have similar but somewhat less problematic proteins.

Long ago humans lived without grain. Today our diets are dominated by it. We eat a muffin for breakfast, a sandwich for lunch and a bowl of pasta for dinner. There's a lot of hidden gluten, soy and corn in processed foods as well. It's used to improve the texture of everything from hot dogs to ketchup. Corn appears as high fructose corn syrup among other manufactured additives. Soy lurks in snack foods, cooking oils and most dairy replacement products. Start reading labels and you will be stunned at the amount of grain you consume without being aware of it.

How About Whole Grains?

Sorry! While whole grains have a better nutritional profile than refined grains, they contain the same anti-nutrients and can cause the same problems.

GRAINS ARE EASY TO SWALLOW, BUT HARD TO DIGEST.

Grain is hard on our digestive system because it contains anti-nutrients. From a plant's perspective these are defensive mechanisms. Plants can't run away from a predator so they evolved chemical protections to make them less attractive as food and to keep them viable. What protects a plant's seeds also protects it from easy digestion, so for humans that makes it an anti-nutrient. One of the many (and most studied) of grains' anti-nutrients is lectin. It occurs in virtually all plants to varying degrees, but is much more concentrated in grain. Lectins are not broken down enough to easily pass into your bloodstream as smaller molecules, so they can compromise the lining of your intestines and cause everything from food intolerances to autoimmune diseases.

WHERE WILL I GET CALCIUM WITHOUT DAIRY?

There are plenty of foods, including dark green leafy vegetables, that supply calcium. More importantly, the body's ability to absorb calcium depends on other nutrients, especially magnesium and vitamin K2, which can come from a variety of vegetable sources. Phytate, an anti-nutrient present in wheat, can also bind with calcium and prevent absorption.

BUT WE NEED CARBS!

Sure we do, but we don't need all the starch and sugar we consume today. We eat a lot more bad carbs than our grandparents did. Carbohydrates are broken down into glucose (sugar) quickly in the bloodstream. If you eat more than you need, your body stores the excess as fat.

There are many sources of good carbs that aren't grain. Fruits and nuts are high in carbohydrates. So are many vegetables including sweet potatoes, carrots and winter squash. They also contribute a wide range of nutrients to your diet.

SAY BYE-BYE TO BEANS

Digesting beans presents most of the same problems as grain. Beans, peanuts (not a nut, but a legume), soybeans and lentils have anti-nutrients just like grains. Like grains, they are difficult to digest. That's why they cause gas. Soaking, fermenting and cooking beans reduces the level of lectins but doesn't remove them. In fact, red kidney beans have such a high concentration of lectin that if they are not thoroughly cooked, they can cause illness. Several outbreaks have been associated with beans prepared in a slow cooker when the temperature was not high enough.

DON'T DO (MOST) DAIRY

Hunter-gatherers certainly didn't have a herd of milk cows following them around. Most of the dairy products we use are highly processed and come from grain-fed cows. They're ultra-pasteurized, homogenized and then fortified to replace nutrients that have been lost. Skim and reduced-fat milk have more lactose, which is milk sugar, because that's what's left when the fat is removed. Lactose intolerance is common. Butter or cream from pasture-raised animals is usually well tolerated since it contains fewer irritating proteins and almost no lactose.

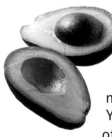

BUT WE NEED FIBER!

Paleo man consumed a great deal of fiber from wild greens and fruits, not from grains or legumes. Following the Paleo path means eating a lot more fruits and vegetables than our modern, grain-heavy diet provides. You'll be getting fiber from avocados, broccoli, carrots and greens instead of a sweet bran muffin or a processed breakfast cereal.

MAKE PALEO FIT YOUR LIFE AND ENJOY WHAT YOU EAT

A healthy diet is one you can stick with for life and that can be tailored to your tastes and sensitivities. Eating Paleo doesn't require counting calories or carbs. How many meals or snacks you have is up to you. Don't sweat it if you break the rules from time to time. This is not a crash diet. Eat whole, natural foods and enjoy them. If you can't live without cheese or the occasional slice of bread, add them in moderation. Once you experience how good it feels to eat the way evolution intended, the rest is easy.

EGGS

CALIFORNIA OMELET WITH AVOCADO

· ·

2 **plum tomatoes, chopped**
2 **to 4 tablespoons chopped fresh cilantro**
½ **teaspoon salt, divided**
8 **eggs**
2 **teaspoons olive oil, divided**
1 **ripe medium avocado, diced**
1 **small cucumber, chopped**

1 Preheat oven to 200°F. Combine tomatoes, cilantro and ¼ teaspoon salt in small bowl; mix well.

2 Whisk eggs and remaining ¼ teaspoon salt in medium bowl until well blended.

3 Heat 1 teaspoon oil in small nonstick skillet over medium heat. Pour half of egg mixture into skillet; cook 2 minutes or until eggs begin to set. Lift edge of omelet to allow uncooked portion to flow underneath. Cook 3 minutes or until set.

4 Spoon half of tomato mixture over half of omelet. Loosen omelet with spatula and fold in half. Slide omelet onto serving plate and keep warm in oven. Repeat with remaining oil, egg mixture and tomato mixture.

5 Cut omelets in half; top with avocado and cucumber; garnish with lemon wedges.

Makes 4 servings

· · · · · · · · · ·

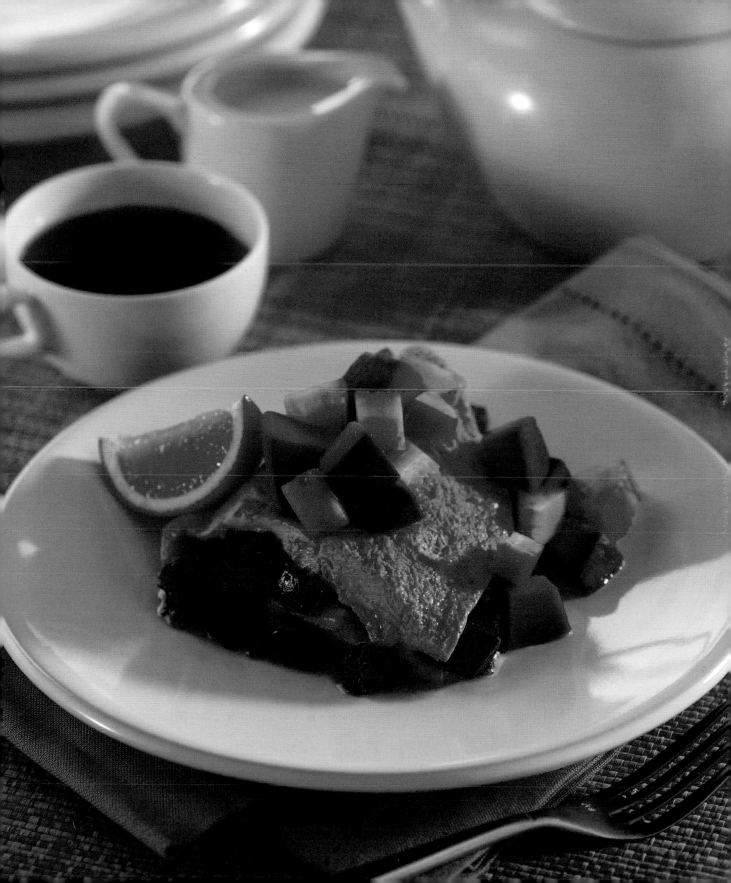

SMOKED SALMON AND SPINACH FRITTATA

- **2 tablespoons olive oil, divided**
- **1 medium red onion, diced**
- **1 clove garlic, minced**
- **6 ounces baby spinach**
- **10 eggs**
- **1 teaspoon dried dill weed**
- **¼ teaspoon salt**
- **¼ teaspoon black pepper**
- **4 ounces smoked salmon, chopped**

1 Preheat broiler.

2 Heat 1 tablespoon oil in large ovenproof nonstick skillet. Add onion; cook 7 to 8 minutes or until softened, stirring occasionally. Add garlic; cook and stir 1 minute. Add spinach; cook 3 minutes or just until wilted. Transfer mixture to small bowl.

3 Whisk eggs, dill, salt and pepper in large bowl until blended. Stir in salmon and spinach mixture.

4 Heat remaining 1 tablespoon oil in same skillet over medium heat. Add egg mixture; cook about 3 minutes, stirring gently to form large curds. Cook without stirring 5 minutes or until eggs are just beginning to set.

5 Transfer skillet to oven; broil 2 to 3 minutes or until frittata is puffed, set and lightly browned. Let stand 5 minutes. Carefully slide frittata onto large plate or cutting board; cut into wedges.

Makes 6 to 8 servings

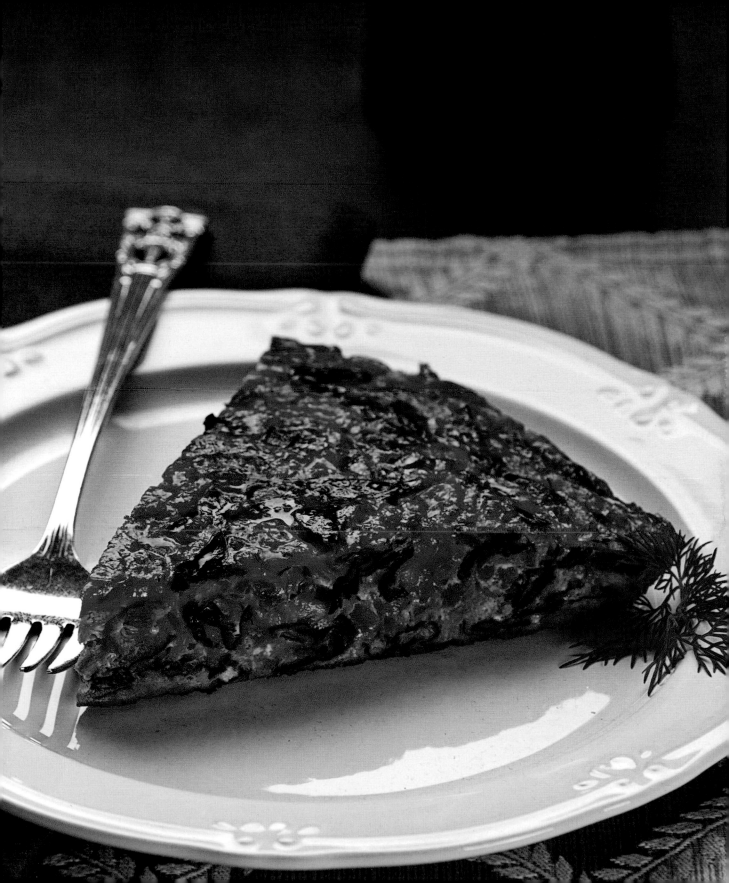

SPICY CRABMEAT FRITTATA

. . . .

  1 **can (about 6 ounces) lump white crabmeat, drained**
  6 **eggs**
 ¼ **teaspoon salt**
 ¼ **teaspoon black pepper**
 ¼ **teaspoon hot pepper sauce**
  1 **tablespoon olive oil**
  1 **green bell pepper, finely chopped**
  2 **cloves garlic, minced**
  1 **plum tomato, seeded and finely chopped**

1 Preheat broiler. Pick out and discard any shell or cartilage from crabmeat; break up large pieces of crabmeat.

2 Whisk eggs in medium bowl. Add crabmeat, salt, black pepper and hot pepper sauce; mix well.

3 Heat oil in large ovenproof skillet over medium-high heat. Add bell pepper and garlic; cook and stir 3 minutes or until tender. Add tomato; cook and stir 1 minute.

4 Reduce heat to medium-low; stir in egg mixture. Cook about 7 minutes or until eggs begin to set around edge of skillet, lifting edge with spatula to allow uncooked portion to flow underneath.

5 Transfer skillet to oven; broil 4 inches from heat source 1 to 2 minutes or until golden brown and center is set.

Makes 4 servings
. . . .

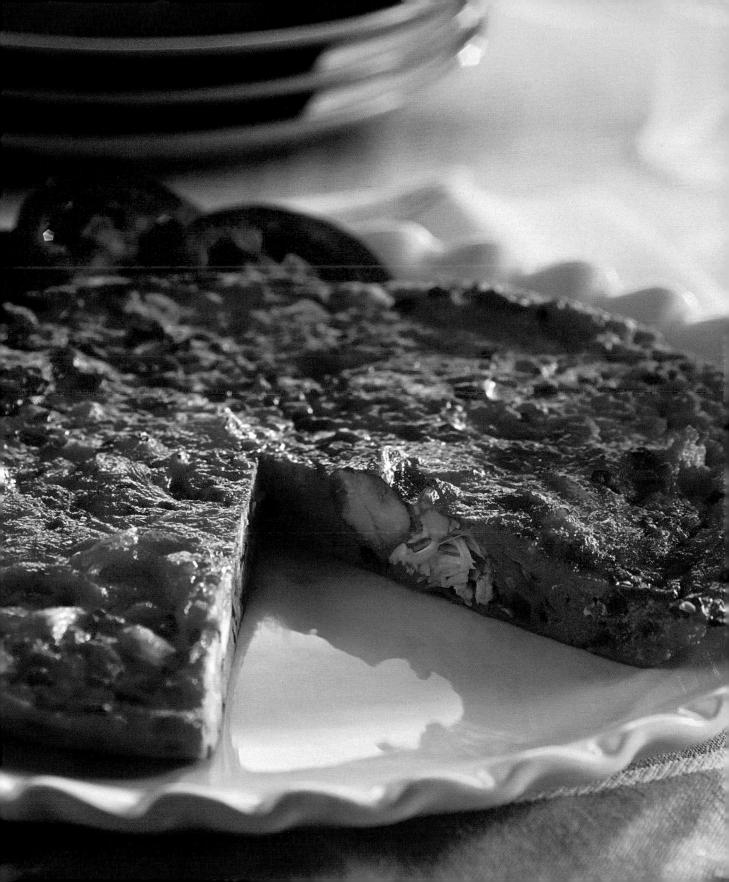

SCOTCH EGGS

· · · · · · · · · ·

1	**pound ground beef or ground turkey**
4	**ounces bulk pork sausage**
⅛	**teaspoon salt**
⅛	**teaspoon black pepper**
1½	**tablespoons olive oil**
6	**hard-cooked eggs, peeled**

1 Preheat oven to 400°F. Spray 11×7-inch baking dish with nonstick cooking spray.

2 Combine beef, sausage, salt and pepper in medium bowl; mix well. Divide mixture into six equal portions.

3 Coat hands lightly with oil. Working with one portion of meat mixture at a time, flatten meat mixture in palm of hand. Place one hard-boiled egg over meat mixture; wrap meat completely around egg. Press meat while turning in hands to completely seal. Brush eggs with remaining oil; place in prepared baking dish.

4 Bake 30 minutes or until meat is cooked through and begins to brown. Cool slightly; cut in half to serve.

Makes 6 servings

· · · · · · · ·

SCRAMBLED EGG AND ZUCCHINI PIE

2 **eggs**
¼ **teaspoon salt**
2 **teaspoons butter**
1 **small zucchini, chopped**

1 Preheat oven to 350°F. Whisk eggs and salt in small bowl until well blended.

2 Melt butter in small nonstick ovenproof skillet over medium-high heat. Add zucchini; cook and stir 2 to 3 minutes or until crisp-tender.

3 Reduce heat to low; stir in egg mixture. Cook without stirring 4 to 5 minutes or until eggs begin to set around edge.

4 Transfer skillet to oven; bake 5 minutes or until eggs are set. Cut into wedges.

Makes 1 serving

THREE-EGG OMELET

3 **eggs**
1 **tablespoon water**
   Salt and black pepper
1 **tablespoon butter**
   Fillings: shredded crabmeat, cooked sliced mushrooms, cooked chopped onion, avocado slices, cooked small shrimp, cooked chopped bell pepper, chopped tomatoes, cooked chopped asparagus and/or cooked chopped broccoli

1 Whisk eggs, water, salt and pepper in small bowl until well blended.

2 Melt butter in small skillet over medium heat. Pour egg mixture into skillet; cook without stirring until egg mixture begins to set. Gently lift cooked edge with spatula to allow uncooked portion to flow underneath. Shake pan several times to loosen omelet. Cook just until set.

3 Place desired fillings on half of omelet. Carefully fold other half over filling. Slide onto serving plate. Serve immediately.

Makes 1 serving

POULTRY

ROAST CHICKEN WITH PEPPERS

- 1 whole chicken (3 to 3½ pounds), cut into pieces
- 3 tablespoons olive oil, divided
- 1½ tablespoons chopped fresh rosemary leaves *or* 1½ teaspoons dried rosemary
- 1 tablespoon lemon juice
- 1¼ teaspoons salt, divided
- ¾ teaspoon black pepper, divided
- 3 bell peppers (red, yellow and/or green)
- 1 medium onion

1 Preheat oven to 375°F. Place chicken in shallow roasting pan.

2 Combine 2 tablespoons oil, rosemary and lemon juice in small bowl; brush over chicken. Sprinkle 1 teaspoon salt and ½ teaspoon black pepper over chicken. Roast 15 minutes.

3 Cut bell peppers into ½-inch strips. Cut onion into thin wedges. Toss vegetables with remaining 1 tablespoon oil, ¼ teaspoon salt and ¼ teaspoon black pepper in medium bowl.

4 Spoon vegetables around chicken; roast about 50 minutes or until vegetables are tender and chicken is cooked through (165°F). Serve chicken with vegetables and pan juices.

Makes 6 servings

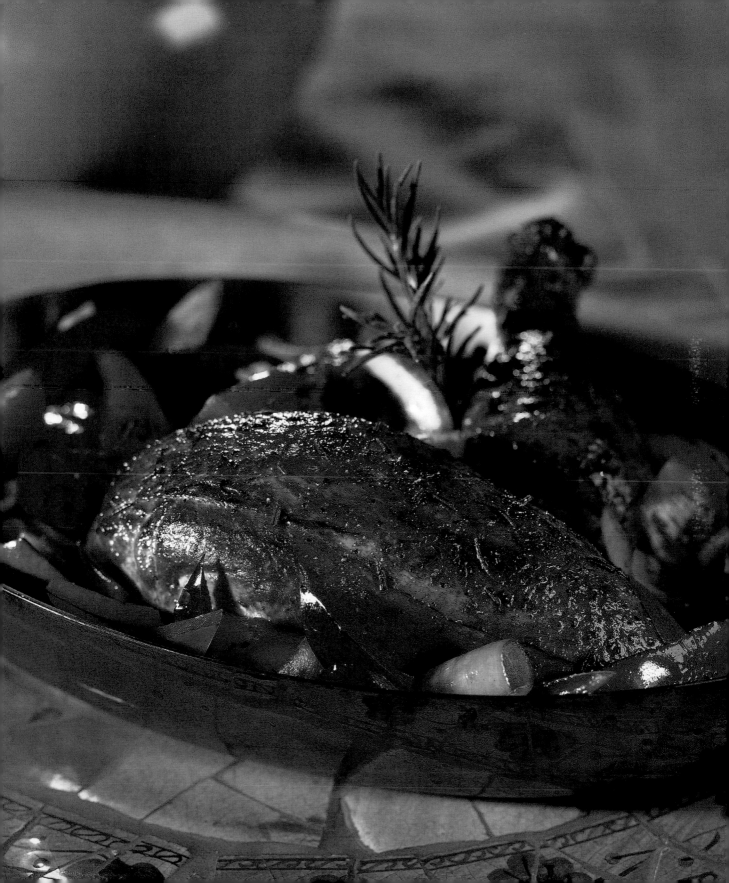

SPICY SQUASH AND CHICKEN SOUP

- 1 tablespoon olive oil
- 1 small onion, finely chopped
- 1 stalk celery, finely chopped
- 2 cups cubed butternut or delicata squash (about 1 small)
- 2 cups chicken broth
- 1 can (about 14 ounces) diced tomatoes with chiles
- 1 cup chopped cooked chicken
- ½ teaspoon salt
- ½ teaspoon ground ginger
- ⅛ teaspoon ground cumin
- ⅛ teaspoon black pepper
- 2 teaspoons lime juice

  Fresh parsley or cilantro sprigs (optional)

1 Heat oil in large saucepan over medium heat. Add onion and celery; cook and stir 5 minutes or just until tender. Stir in squash, broth, tomatoes, chicken, salt, ginger, cumin and pepper.

2 Cover and cook over low heat 30 minutes or until squash is tender. Stir in lime juice. Sprinkle with parsley.

Makes 4 servings

TIP: Butternut and delicata are two types of winter squash. Butternut is a long, light orange squash. Delicata is an elongated, creamy yellow squash with green striations. Both have hard skins. To use, cut the squash lengthwise, scoop out the seeds, peel and cut into cubes.

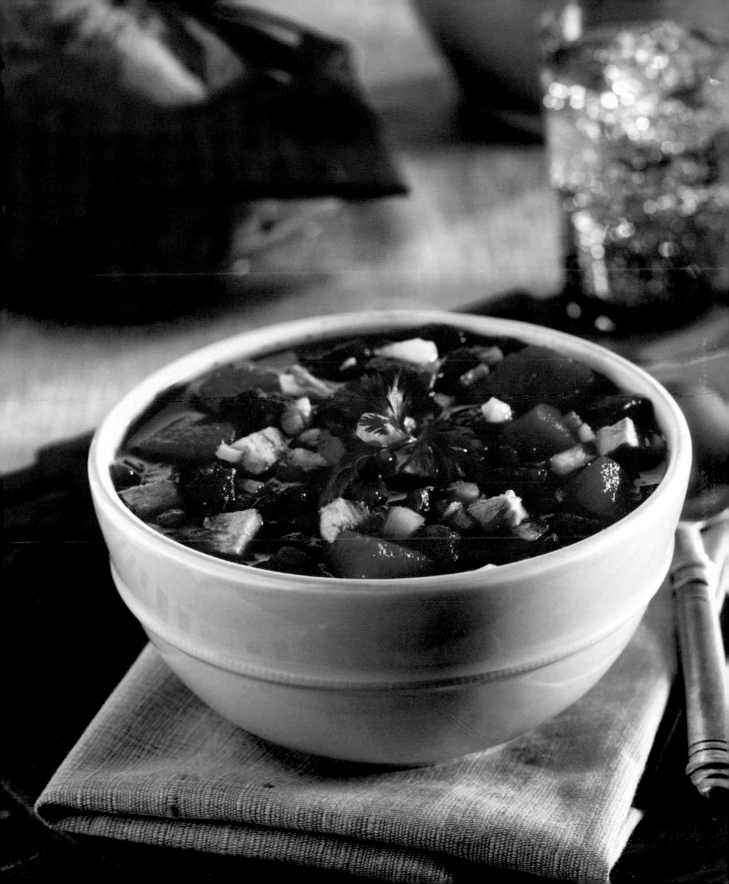

GRILLED CHICKEN ADOBO

· · · · · · · · · · · · · · · ·

½ **cup chopped onion**
⅓ **cup lime juice**
6 **cloves garlic, coarsely chopped**
1 **teaspoon ground cumin**
1 **teaspoon dried oregano**
½ **teaspoon dried thyme**
¼ **teaspoon ground red pepper**
6 **boneless skinless chicken breasts (about 4 ounces each)**
3 **tablespoons chopped fresh cilantro (optional)**

1 Combine onion, lime juice and garlic in food processor; process until onion is finely minced. Transfer to resealable food storage bag.

2 Add cumin, oregano, thyme and red pepper; knead bag until blended. Add chicken to bag. Seal bag; turn to coat. Marinate in refrigerator 30 minutes or up to 4 hours, turning occasionally.

3 Oil grid. Prepare grill for direct cooking. Remove chicken from marinade; discard marinade.

4 Grill chicken over medium heat 5 to 7 minutes per side or until no longer pink in center. Garnish with cilantro, if desired.

Makes 6 servings

· · · · · · · ·

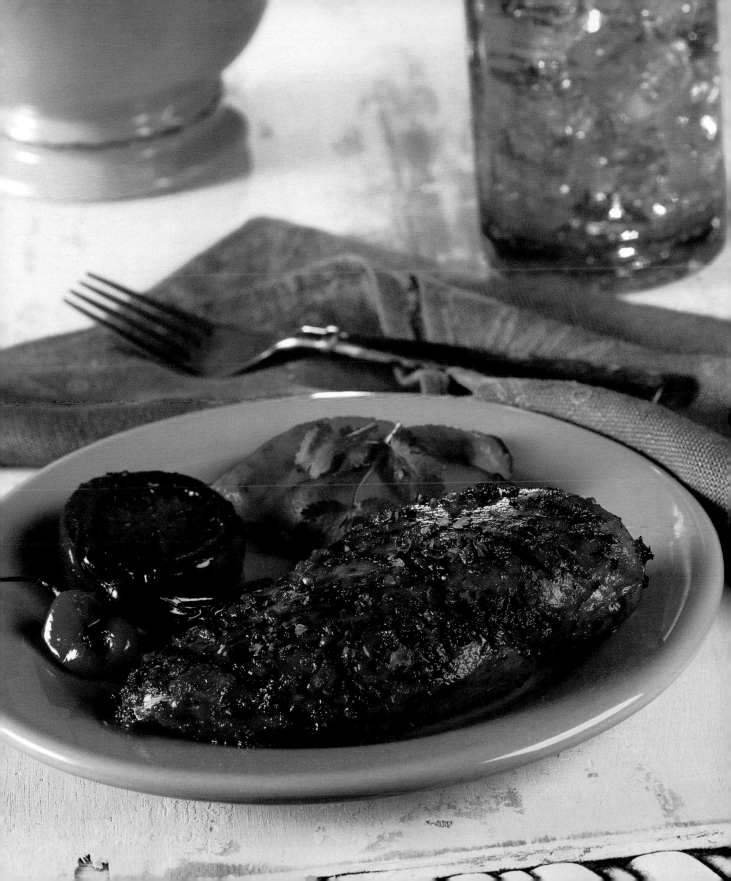

CHICKEN MIRABELLA

. . . .

  4 **boneless skinless chicken breasts (about 4 ounces each)**
 ½ **cup pitted prunes**
 ½ **cup assorted pitted olives (black, green and/or a combination)**
 ¼ **cup white wine**
  2 **tablespoons olive oil**
  1 **tablespoon capers**
  1 **tablespoon red wine vinegar**
  1 **teaspoon dried oregano**
  1 **clove garlic, minced**
  1 **teaspoon chopped fresh parsley**
  2 **teaspoons honey**

1 Preheat oven to 350°F.

2 Place chicken in 8-inch square baking dish. Combine prunes, olives, wine, oil, capers, vinegar, oregano, garlic and parsley in medium bowl. Pour mixture over chicken; drizzle with honey.

3 Bake 25 to 30 minutes or until chicken is no longer pink in center, basting with sauce halfway through cooking time.

Makes 4 servings

. . . .

TIP: For more intense flavor, marinate chicken 8 hours or overnight

TURKEY LETTUCE WRAPS

- 1 teaspoon dark sesame oil
- 1 pound ground turkey
- ½ cup sliced green onions
- 2 tablespoons minced fresh ginger
- 1 can (8 ounces) water chestnuts, chopped
- 1 teaspoon coconut aminos*
- ¼ cup chopped fresh cilantro
- 12 large lettuce leaves
  Chopped fresh mint leaves (optional)

*Coconut aminos is a dark, salty soy-free sauce containing 17 amino acids. It is made from the sap of the coconut tree which is dried and blended with sea salt. It does not have a pronounced coconut flavor and is often used as a substitute for soy sauce in paleo recipes. Coconut aminos can be found in health food and vitamin stores, some grocery stores or online.

1 Heat oil in large skillet over medium-high heat. Add turkey, green onions and ginger; cook 6 to 8 minutes, stirring to break up meat.

2 Add water chestnuts and coconut aminos to skillet; cook and stir 3 minutes or until turkey is cooked through. Remove from heat; stir in cilantro.

3 Spoon ¼ cup turkey mixture onto each lettuce leaf. Top with mint, if desired. Roll up to enclose filling.

Makes 12 wraps (about 6 servings)

HONEY-ROASTED CHICKEN AND BUTTERNUT SQUASH

1 **pound peeled seeded butternut squash chunks**
1 **tablespoon plus 1 teaspoon olive oil, divided**
Salt and black pepper
6 **bone-in chicken thighs**
1 **tablespoon honey**

1 Preheat oven to 375°F.

2 Place squash on large baking sheet. Drizzle with 1 tablespoon oil and season with salt and pepper; toss to coat. Spread in single layer.

3 Place wire rack over squash; brush with remaining 1 teaspoon oil. Arrange chicken on rack; season with salt and pepper.

4 Roast 25 minutes. Carefully lift rack and stir squash; brush honey over chicken. Roast 20 minutes or until chicken is cooked through (165°F).

Makes 4 to 6 servings

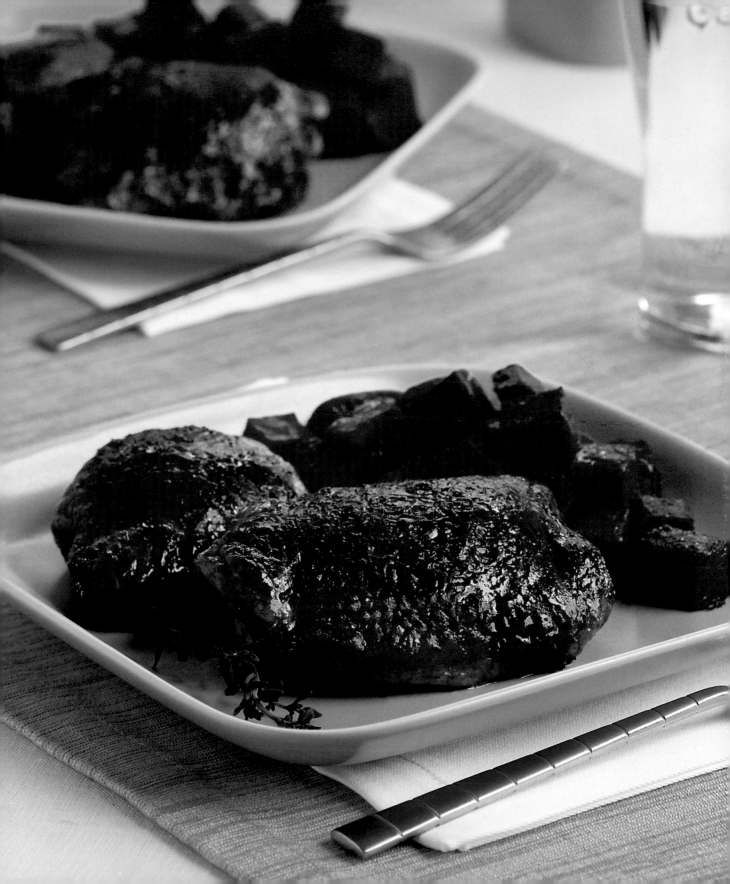

LEMON CHICKEN

- 2 tablespoons extra virgin olive oil, divided
- 4 boneless skinless chicken breasts (4 ounces each) flattened to ½-inch thickness
- 1 cup sliced mushrooms
- ½ cup white wine
  Juice of 1 lemon
- 2 tablespoons capers
- 1 teaspoon chopped fresh dill, plus additional for garnish
- ¼ teaspoon salt
  Lemon wedges (optional)

1 Heat 1 tablespoon oil in large nonstick skillet over medium-high heat. Add chicken; cook 3 to 4 minutes or until chicken begins to brown.

2 Meanwhile, combine mushrooms, wine, lemon juice, capers, dill and salt in medium bowl; mix well.

3 Turn chicken; pour mushroom mixture evenly over chicken. Reduce heat to medium-low; cover and simmer 8 minutes or until chicken is no longer pink in center.

4 Remove chicken to serving platter; cover to keep warm. Increase heat to medium-high; boil liquid in skillet 1 minute to reduce slightly. Remove from heat; stir in remaining 1 tablespoon oil. Garnish with additional dill and lemon wedges, if desired.

Makes 4 servings

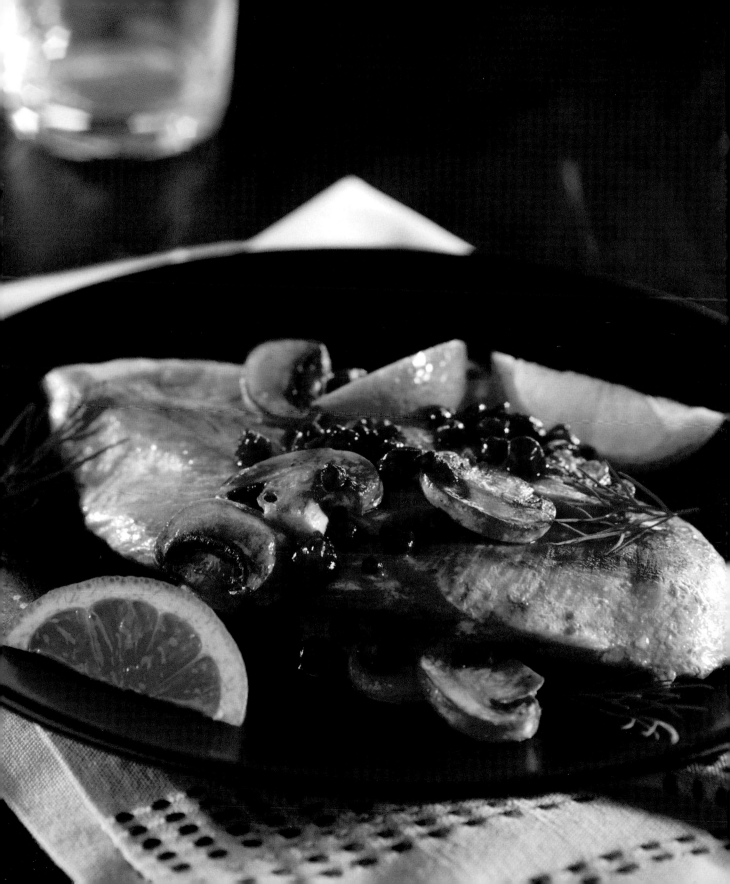

JERK TURKEY STEW

- 1 tablespoon olive oil
- 1 small red onion, chopped
- 1 clove garlic, minced
- ½ teaspoon salt
- ½ teaspoon ground ginger
- ¼ teaspoon black pepper
- ⅛ to ¼ teaspoon ground red pepper*
- ⅛ teaspoon ground allspice
- 1 can (about 28 ounces) diced tomatoes
- 3 cups diced cooked turkey
- 2 cups cooked sweet potato (½-inch pieces)
- ½ cup turkey or chicken broth
- 1 tablespoon lime juice
- 1 tablespoon minced fresh chives

1 Heat oil in large saucepan or Dutch oven over medium heat. Add onion and garlic; cook and stir 5 minutes. Add salt, ginger, black pepper, red pepper and allspice; cook and stir 1 minute.

2 Stir in tomatoes, turkey, sweet potato and broth; bring to a boil over high heat. Reduce heat to low; simmer 15 minutes.

3 Stir in lime juice; cover and let stand 10 minutes. Sprinkle with chives just before serving.

Makes 4 servings

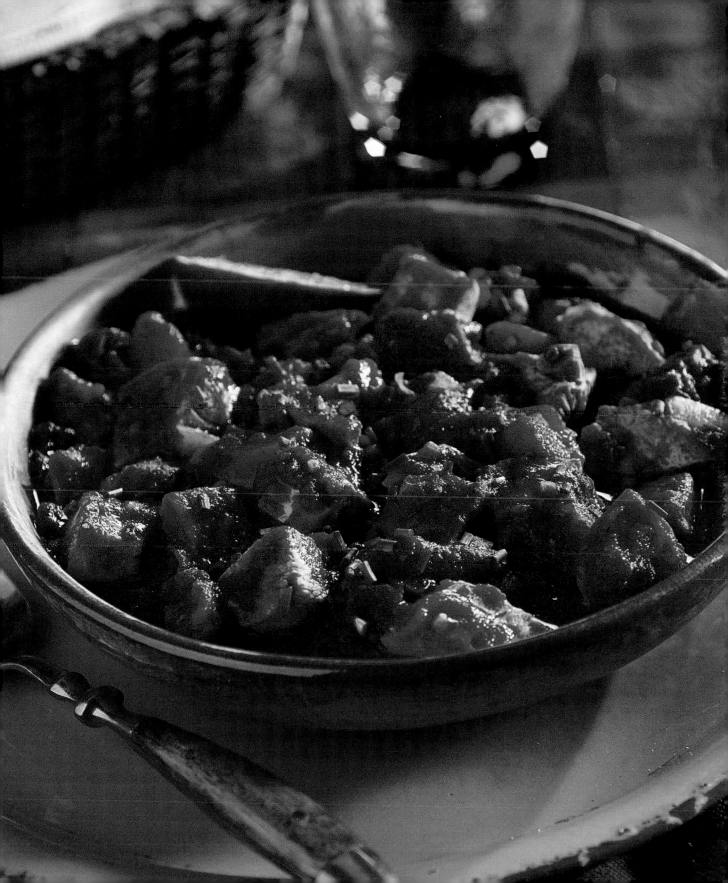

JALAPEÑO-LIME CHICKEN

- 1 tablespoon olive oil
- 1 tablespoon lime juice
- 1 jalapeño pepper,* seeded and diced
- 1 teaspoon ground cumin
- 1 teaspoon grated lime peel
- 2 cloves garlic, minced
- ½ teaspoon salt
- 1 pound boneless skinless chicken breasts
  Sliced jalapeño peppers* and black olives (optional)

Jalapeño peppers can sting and irritate the skin, so wear rubber gloves when handling peppers and do not touch your eyes.

1 Combine oil, lime juice, jalapeño, cumin, lime peel, garlic and salt in small bowl; mix well. Brush mixture on both sides of chicken. Cover and marinate in refrigerator 30 minutes or up to 8 hours.

2 Oil grid. Prepare grill for direct cooking.

3 Grill chicken over medium-high heat 5 to 6 minutes per side or until no longer pink in center. Garnish with sliced jalapeños and black olives, if desired.

Makes 4 servings

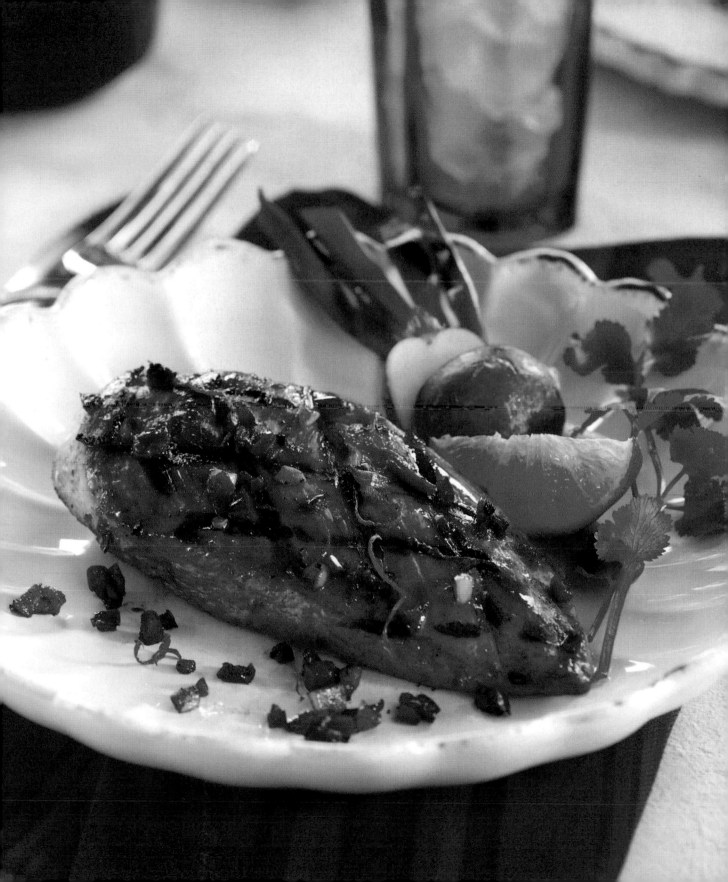

ROASTED ROSEMARY CHICKEN LEGS

¼ cup finely chopped onion
2 tablespoons butter, melted
1 tablespoon chopped fresh rosemary leaves *or* 1 teaspoon dried rosemary
2 cloves garlic, minced
½ teaspoon salt
¼ teaspoon black pepper
4 chicken legs (about 1½ pounds)
¼ cup white wine or chicken broth

1 Preheat oven to 375°F.

2 Combine onion, butter, rosemary, garlic, salt and pepper in small bowl; mix well. Gently loosen chicken skin; rub onion mixture under and over skin. Place chicken, skin side up, in small shallow roasting pan. Pour wine over chicken.

3 Roast chicken 50 to 60 minutes or until chicken is browned and cooked through (165°F), basting frequently with pan juices.

Makes 4 servings

VEGGIE-PACKED TURKEY BURGERS

1¼ pounds ground turkey
½ cup chopped onion
½ cup shredded zucchini
½ cup shredded carrot
1 teaspoon minced jalapeño pepper
Salt and black pepper
Shredded lettuce and tomato slices

1 Oil grid. Prepare grill for direct cooking. Combine turkey, onion, zucchini, carrot, jalapeño, salt and black pepper in large bowl. Shape into four patties.

2 Grill, covered, over medium-heat 8 to 10 minutes or until cooked through (160°F), turning halfway through grilling. Serve with lettuce and tomato.

Makes 4 servings

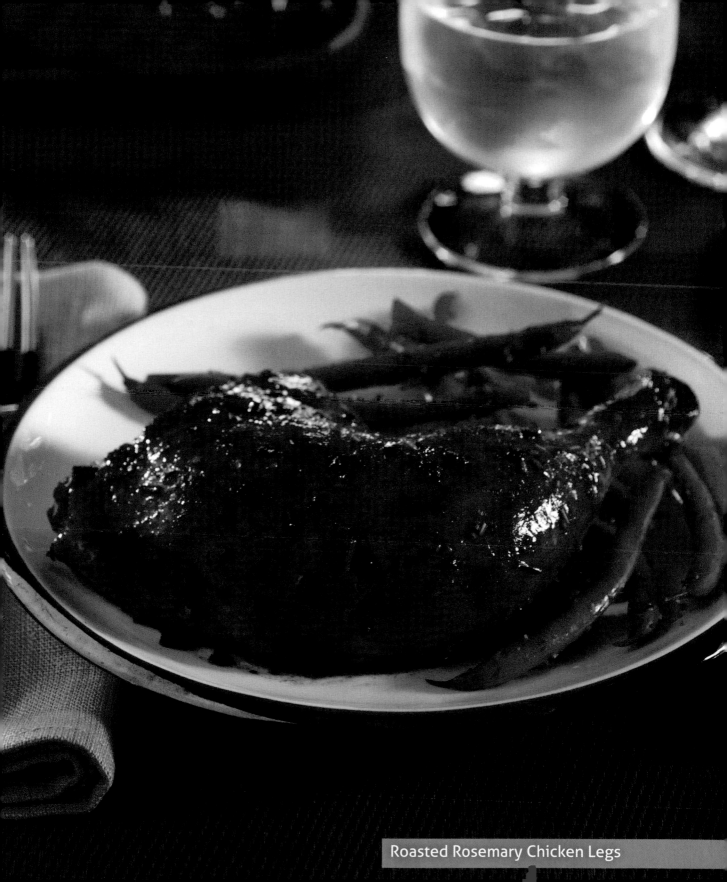

Roasted Rosemary Chicken Legs

BALSAMIC CHICKEN

· · · · · · · · · · · · · ·

  1½ teaspoons fresh rosemary leaves, minced *or* ½ teaspoon dried rosemary
   2 cloves garlic, minced
   ¾ teaspoon black pepper
   ½ teaspoon salt
   6 boneless skinless chicken breasts (about 4 ounces each)
  1½ tablespoons olive oil, divided
   ¼ cup balsamic vinegar

1 Combine rosemary, garlic, pepper and salt in small bowl; mix well. Place chicken in large bowl; drizzle with 1 tablespoon oil and rub with spice mixture. Cover and refrigerate 2 to 3 hours.

2 Preheat oven to 450°F. Brush heavy roasting pan or cast iron skillet with remaining ½ tablespoon oil. Place chicken in pan; bake 10 minutes. Turn chicken, stirring in 3 to 4 tablespoons water if drippings begin to stick to pan.

3 Bake about 10 minutes or until chicken is golden brown and no longer pink in center. If pan is dry, stir in 1 to 2 tablespoons water to loosen drippings.

4 Drizzle vinegar over chicken in pan. Transfer chicken to plates. Stir liquid in pan, scraping up browned bits. Drizzle over chicken.

Makes 6 servings

· · · · · · · ·

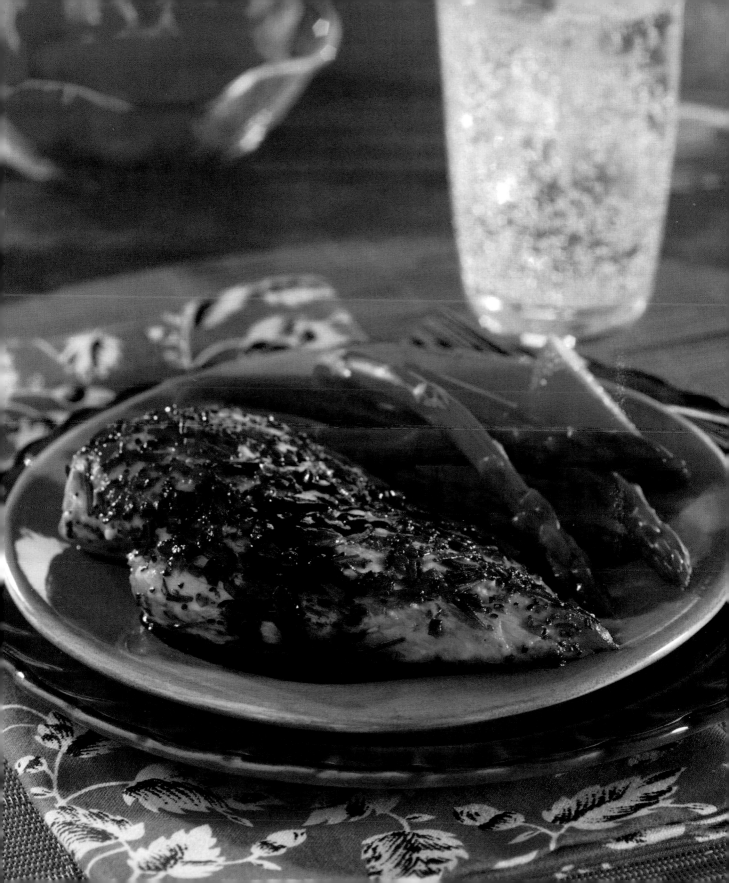

SWEET SPICED TARRAGON ROAST TURKEY BREAST

- 2 tablespoons plus 1 teaspoon olive oil, divided
- 2 teaspoons grated orange peel
- 1½ teaspoons dried tarragon
- 1 teaspoon ground cumin
- ½ teaspoon salt
- ½ teaspoon ground allspice
- ½ teaspoon ground cinnamon
- ½ teaspoon ground ginger
- ½ teaspoon black pepper
- ¼ teaspoon ground red pepper
- 1 (2½-pound) bone-in turkey breast half, thawed if frozen

1 Preheat oven to 400°F. Brush broiler pan with 1 teaspoon oil.

2 Combine remaining 2 tablespoons oil, orange peel, tarragon, cumin, salt, allspice, cinnamon, ginger, black pepper and red pepper in small bowl; mix well. Gently loosen skin from turkey; rub tarragon mixture under skin. Place turkey, skin side up, in prepared pan.

3 Roast 1 hour and 15 minutes or until cooked through (165°F). Cover loosely and let stand 15 minutes. Cut turkey into thin slices.

Makes 4 to 6 servings

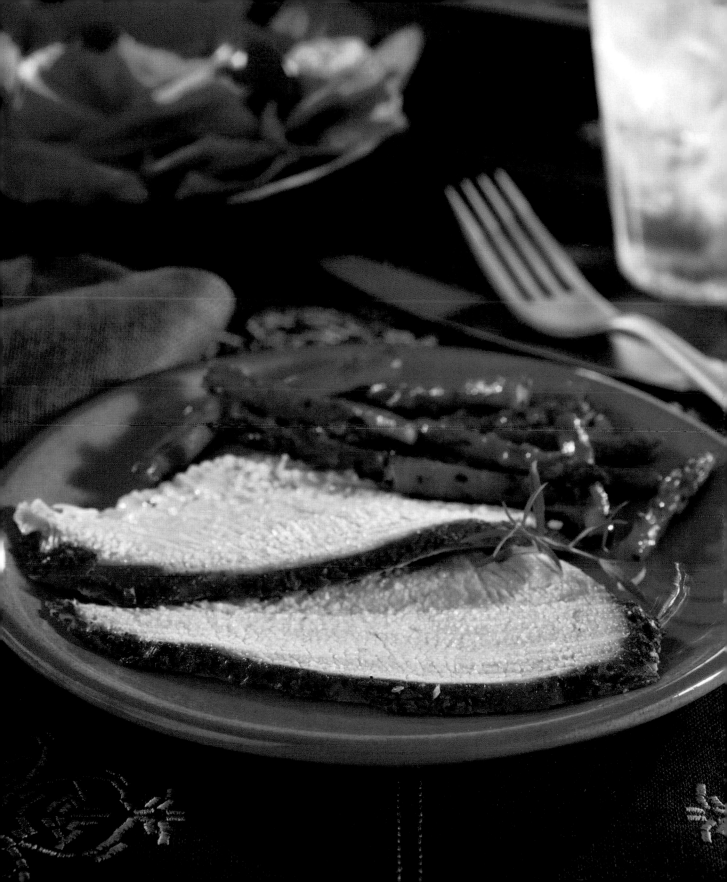

CURRIED CHICKEN AND WINTER VEGETABLE STEW

1 tablespoon olive oil

1 pound boneless skinless chicken breasts, cut into ½-inch cubes

1 tablespoon curry powder

3½ cups chicken broth

1 can (about 14 ounces) diced tomatoes

2 medium turnips, cut into 1-inch pieces

2 medium carrots, halved lengthwise, then cut crosswise into 1-inch slices

1 medium onion, chopped

¼ cup tomato paste

½ cup raisins (optional)

½ teaspoon salt

½ teaspoon black pepper

1 Heat oil in large saucepan over medium heat. Add chicken; cook and stir 5 minutes or until lightly browned. Add curry powder; cook and stir 1 minute.

2 Stir in broth, tomatoes, turnips, carrots, onion, tomato paste, raisins, if desired, salt and pepper; bring to a boil. Reduce heat to low; cover and simmer 15 minutes or until vegetables are tender, stirring occasionally.

Makes 6 servings

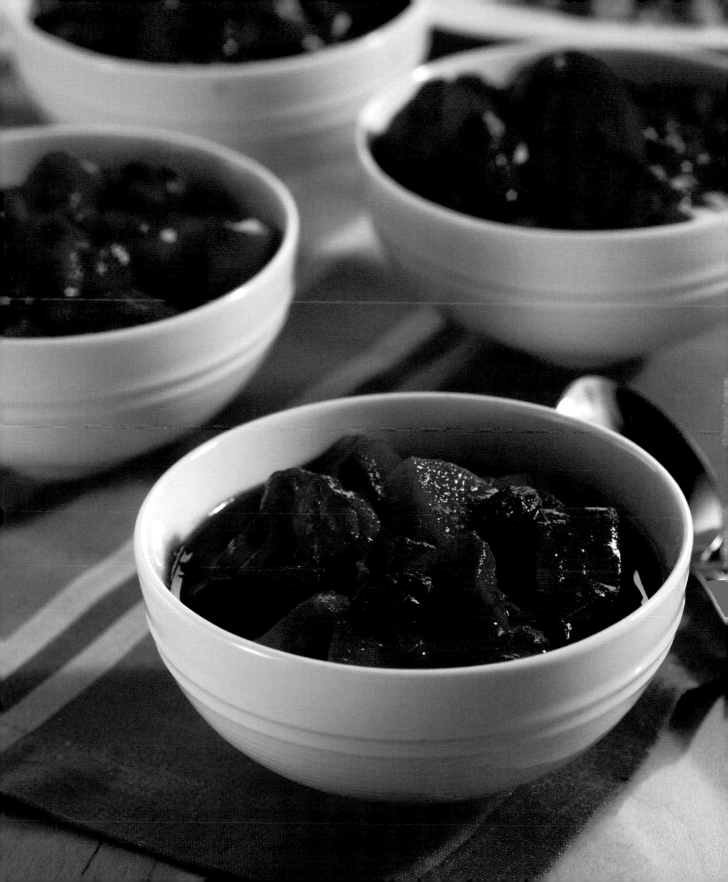

GREEK ROAST CHICKEN

- 1 whole roasting chicken (4 to 5 pounds)
- 3 tablespoons olive oil, divided
- 2 tablespoons chopped fresh rosemary leaves, plus fresh sprigs
- 2 cloves garlic, minced
- 1 lemon
- 1¼ teaspoons salt, divided
- ½ teaspoon black pepper, divided
- 1¾ cups chicken broth or stock, divided
- 2 large sweet potatoes, peeled and cut into thick wedges
- 1 medium red onion, cut into ¼-inch wedges
- 1 pound asparagus, trimmed

1 Preheat oven to 425°F. Place chicken, breast side up, in shallow roasting pan.

2 Combine 2 tablespoons oil, chopped rosemary and garlic in small bowl; brush over chicken.

3 Grate 1 teaspoon peel from lemon; set aside. Cut lemon into quarters; squeeze juice over chicken and place lemon quarters and rosemary sprigs in cavity. Sprinkle chicken with ¾ teaspoon salt and ¼ teaspoon pepper. Pour 1 cup broth into bottom of roasting pan; roast 30 minutes.

4 *Reduce oven temperature to 375°F.* Arrange sweet potatoes and onion wedges in single layer around chicken in roasting pan. Drizzle remaining ¾ cup broth and 1 tablespoon oil over vegetables; roast 15 minutes.

5 Arrange asparagus in roasting pan; sprinkle with remaining ½ teaspoon salt and ¼ teaspoon pepper. Roast 10 minutes or until chicken is cooked through (165°F) and vegetables are tender. Transfer chicken to cutting board. Tent with foil; let stand 10 to 15 minutes.

6 Sprinkle reserved lemon peel over chicken. Serve with vegetables and pan juices.

Makes 8 servings

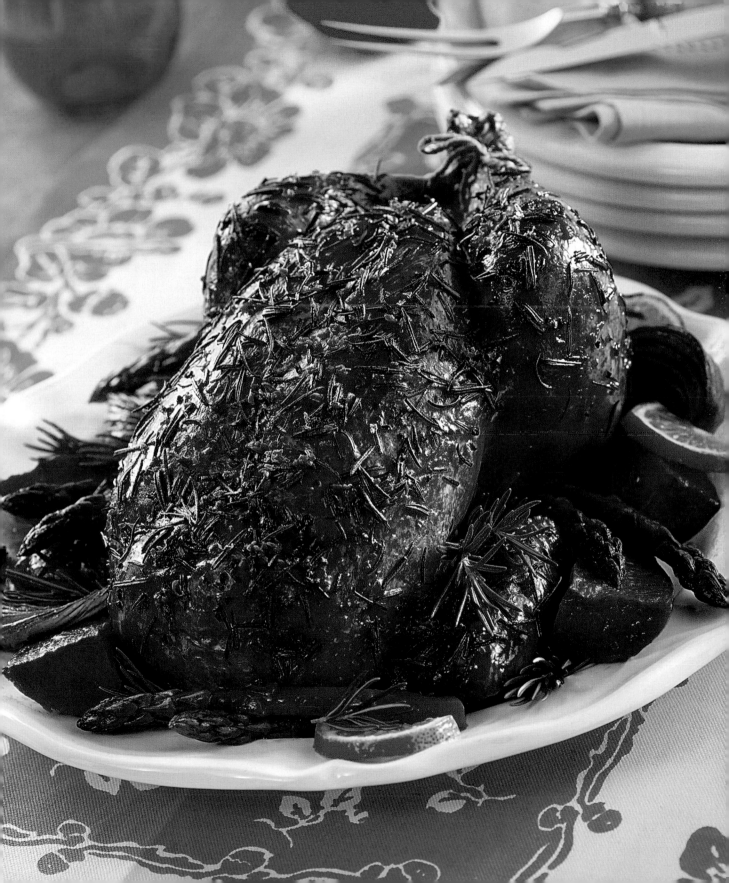

ROAST CHICKEN AND OLIVE KABOBS

- 3 tablespoons olive oil
- 1 tablespoon lemon juice
- ¼ teaspoon salt
- ¼ teaspoon dried oregano
- ¼ teaspoon red pepper flakes
- ¼ teaspoon paprika
- ⅛ teaspoon black pepper
- 3 boneless skinless chicken thighs (about 8 ounces), each cut into 4 pieces
- 12 large pitted green olives

1 Combine oil, lemon juice, salt, oregano, red pepper flakes, paprika and black pepper in small bowl; mix well. Add chicken; stir to coat. Cover and refrigerate 2 to 3 hours, turning chicken once.

2 Preheat oven to 425°F. Remove chicken from marinade; discard marinade. Alternately thread chicken and olives onto six metal skewers. Place kabobs on rack in shallow baking pan.

3 Roast 15 to 18 minutes or until chicken is cooked through, turning halfway through cooking time.

Makes 4 servings

SOUTHWEST CHICKEN BURGERS
WITH AVOCADO SALAD

- 1 cup finely diced yellow or red bell pepper, divided
- ½ cup finely diced red onion, divided
- 1 egg
- 1½ teaspoons chili powder, divided
- ¾ teaspoon salt, divided
- 1¼ pounds ground chicken
- 1 medium avocado, diced
- ½ cup finely diced cucumber
- Juice of 1 lime
- 1 tablespoon olive oil

1 For burgers, combine ½ cup bell pepper, ¼ cup onion, egg, 1 teaspoon chili powder and ½ teaspoon salt in large bowl. Add chicken; stir gently until blended. Shape mixture into six patties. Cover and refrigerate 15 minutes.

2 For salad, combine avocado, cucumber, lime juice, remaining ½ cup bell pepper, ¼ cup onion, ½ teaspoon chili powder and ¼ teaspoon salt in medium bowl; toss gently.

3 Heat oil in large skillet over medium heat. Add burgers; cook 5 minutes per side or until cooked through (165°F).

4 Divide avocado salad among four plates; top with burgers.

Makes 6 servings

CHUNKY CHICKEN STEW

- 1 tablespon olive oil
- 1 small onion, chopped
- 1 cup thinly sliced carrots
- 1 chicken broth
- 1 can (about 14 ounces) diced tomatoes
- 1 cup diced cooked chicken breast
- 3 cups sliced kale or baby spinach
  Salt and black pepper

1 Heat oil in large saucepan over medium-high heat. Add onion; cook and stir about 7 minutes or until golden brown. Stir in carrots and broth; bring to a boil. Reduce heat to low; simmer, uncovered, 5 minutes.

2 Stir in tomatoes; simmer 5 minutes or until carrots are tender. Add chicken; cook and stir until heated through. Add kale; stir until wilted. Season with salt and pepper.

Makes 2 servings

GINGER-LIME CHICKEN THIGHS

- ⅓ cup olive oil
- 3 tablespoons *each* lime juice and honey
- 2 teaspoons grated fresh ginger *or* 1 teaspoon ground ginger
- ½ teaspoon salt
- ¼ to ½ teaspoon red pepper flakes
- 6 boneless skinless chicken thighs

1 Combine oil, lime juice, honey, ginger, salt and red pepper flakes in small bowl. Place chicken in large resealable food storage bag. Add ½ cup marinade; reserve remaining marinade. Seal bag; turn to coat. Marinate in refrigerator 30 minutes, turning occasionally.

2 Oil grid. Prepare grill for direct cooking.

3 Remove chicken from marinade; discard marinade. Grill chicken over medium-high heat 12 minutes or until chicken is no longer pink in center, turning once. Brush with reserved marinade during last 5 minutes of grilling.

Makes 2 to 4 servings

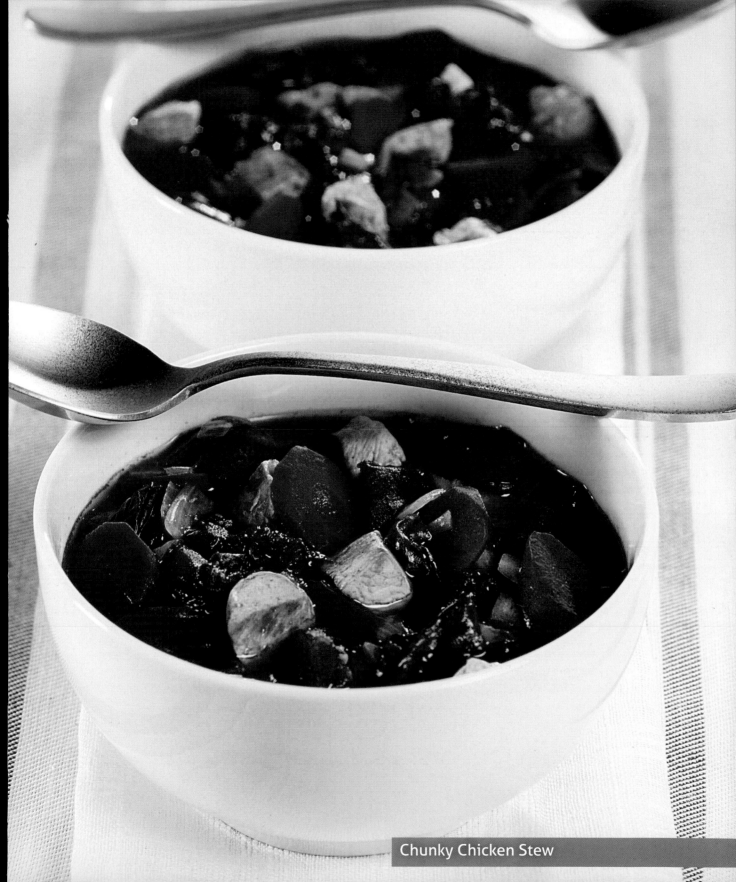

Chunky Chicken Stew

BEEF

BEEF TENDERLOIN WITH HIGH SPICE RUB

- 1 tablespoon onion powder
- 2 teaspoons dried thyme
- 1 teaspoon ground cumin
- ¾ teaspoon ground allspice
- 1 teaspoon black pepper or lemon pepper
- ⅛ teaspoon ground red pepper
- ½ teaspoon salt
- 2 pounds beef tenderloin
- 1 tablespoon olive oil
- ¼ cup water

1 Combine onion powder, thyme, cumin, allspice, black pepper, red pepper and salt in small bowl. Sprinkle evenly over all sides of beef, pressing down firmly so seasonings will adhere. Wrap tightly with plastic wrap; refrigerate 24 hours.

2 Preheat oven to 400°F. Line large rimmed baking pan with foil. Heat oil in large skillet over medium-high heat. Add beef; cook 5 minutes or until well browned, turning once. Transfer beef to prepared pan. Add water to skillet; cook 15 seconds, scraping up browned bits from bottom of skillet. Drizzle over beef.

3 Roast, uncovered, 25 minutes until 135°F or until desired doneness. Tent with foil; let stand 10 minutes. Slice beef; drizzle with pan drippings.

Makes 6 to 8 servings

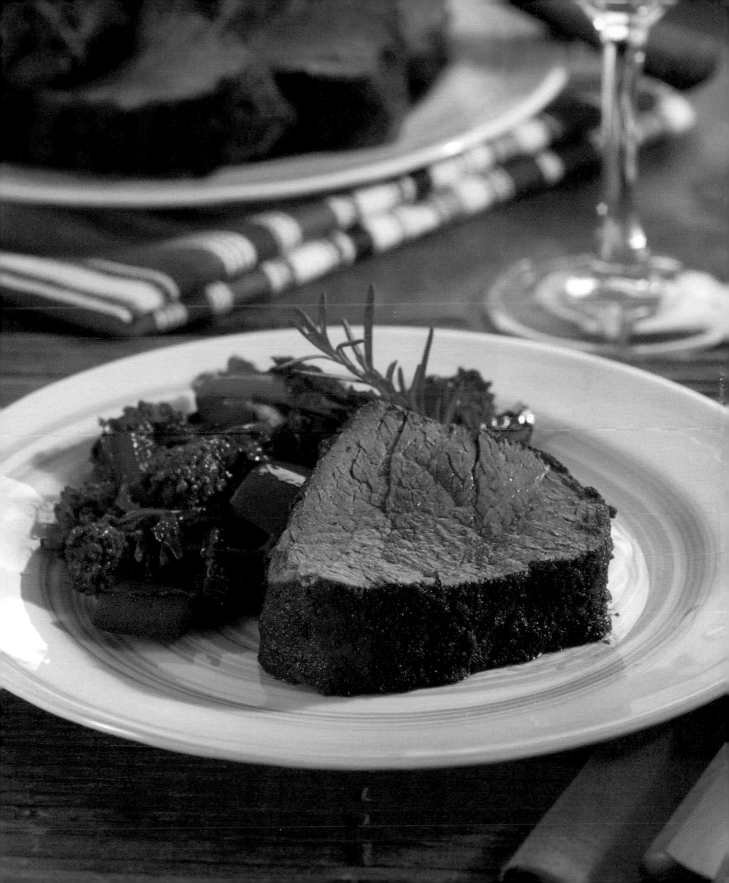

MUSTARD CRUSTED RIB ROAST

　1　**(3-rib) beef rib roast, trimmed* (6 to 7 pounds)**
　3　**tablespoons Dijon mustard**
1½　**tablespoons chopped fresh tarragon** *or* **1½ teaspoons dried tarragon**
　3　**cloves garlic, minced**
　¼　**cup dry red wine**
　⅓　**cup finely chopped shallots (about 2 shallots)**
　1　**cup beef broth**

*Ask butcher to remove chine bone for easier carving. Trim fat to ¼-inch thickness.

1 Preheat oven to 450°F. Place roast, bone side down, in shallow roasting pan. Combine mustard, tarragon and garlic in small bowl; spread over all surfaces of roast except bottom. Roast 10 minutes.

2 *Reduce oven temperature to 350°F.* Roast 2½ to 3 hours until 140°F for medium or until desired doneness.

3 Transfer roast to cutting board; tent with foil. Let stand 10 to 15 minutes before carving. (Internal temperature will continue to rise 5°F to 10°F during stand time.)

4 Reserve 1 tablespoon drippings from roasting pan in medium saucepan; discard remaining drippings. Add wine to roasting pan; place over two burners. Cook over medium heat 2 minutes or until slightly thickened, scraping up browned bits from bottom of pan.

5 Add shallots to reserved drippings in saucepan; cook and stir over medium heat 4 minutes or until softened. Add broth and wine mixture; cook about 8 minutes or until sauce reduces slightly, stirring occasionally. Strain through fine-mesh strainer before serving.

6 Carve roast into ½-inch-thick slices. Serve with sauce.

Makes 6 to 8 servings

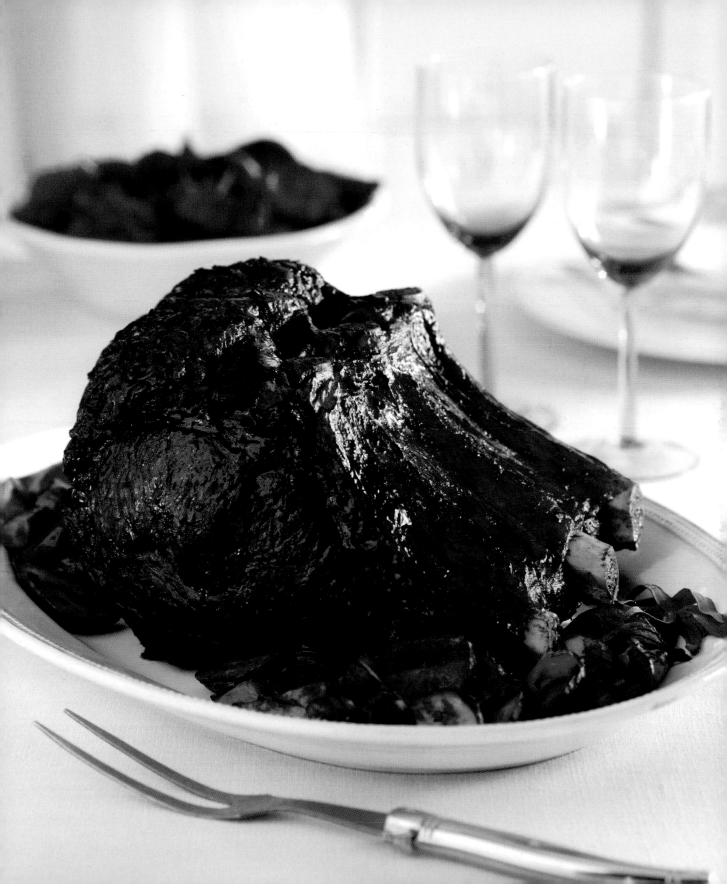

WARM STEAK SALAD WITH MUSTARD DRESSING

Mustard Dressing (recipe follows)
1 beef flank steak (about 1¼ pounds)
Salt and black pepper
¼ pound sugar snap peas or snow peas
Lettuce leaves
1 medium red onion, sliced, separated into rings
1 pint cherry tomatoes

1 Preheat broiler. Position oven rack 4 inches from heat source. Prepare Mustard Dressing; set aside.

2 Place steak on rack of broiler pan. Broil 13 to 18 minutes for medium-rare to medium or until desired doneness, turning once. Season with salt and pepper. Let stand 5 minutes.

3 Meanwhile, bring lightly salted water to a boil in medium saucepan over medium heat. Add snap peas; cook 2 minutes. Drain.

4 Cut steak across the grain into thin slices. Serve with onion, tomatoes and snap peas. Serve with dressing.

Makes 4 servings

MUSTARD DRESSING

¾ cup olive oil
3 tablespoons rice vinegar
1 tablespoon balsamic vinegar
1 tablespoon Dijon mustard*
¼ teaspoon dried thyme leaves
Salt and black pepper

Or substitute coarse-grain mustard for Dijon mustard.

Combine oil, rice vinegar, balsamic vinegar, mustard and thyme in small bowl; mix well. Season with salt and pepper.

Makes about 1 cup

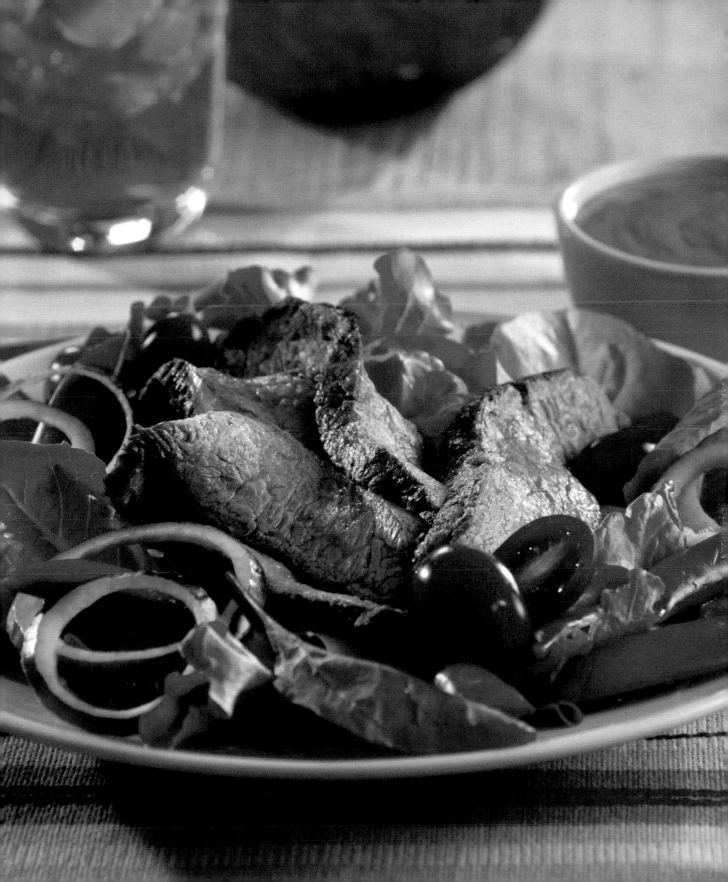

CHILI Á LA MEXICO

  2 pounds ground beef
  2 cups finely chopped onions
  2 cloves garlic, minced
  1 can (28 ounces) whole peeled tomatoes, undrained, coarsely chopped
  1 can (6 ounces) tomato paste
1½ to 2 tablespoons chili powder
  1 teaspoon ground cumin
  ¼ teaspoon salt
  ¼ teaspoon ground red pepper
  ¼ teaspoon ground cloves (optional)
     Lime wedges and fresh cilantro (optional)

1 Brown beef in deep skillet over medium-high heat 6 to 8 minutes, stirring to separate meat. Drain fat. Add onions and garlic to skillet; cook and stir over medium heat 5 minutes or until onions are softened.

2 Stir in tomatoes with juice, tomato paste, chili powder, cumin, salt, red pepper and cloves, if desired; bring to a boil over high heat. Reduce heat to low; cover and simmer 30 minutes, stirring occasionally. Garnish with lime and cilantro.

Makes 6 to 8 servings

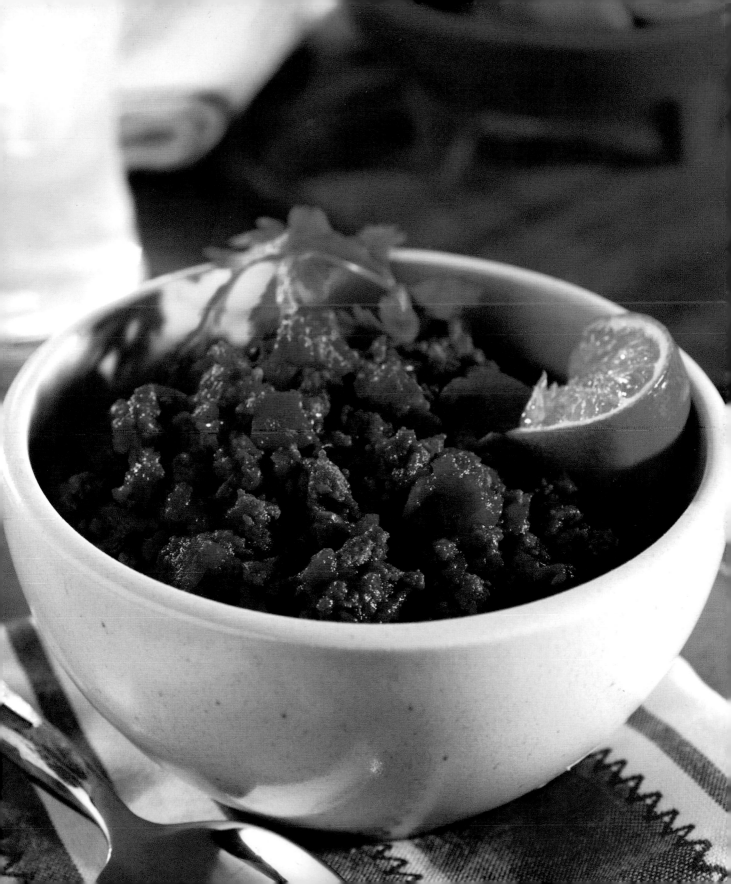

BEEF POT ROAST

- 1 tablespoon olive oil
- 1 beef eye of round roast (about 2½ pounds), trimmed
- 1½ cups beef broth
- 2 cloves garlic
- 1 teaspoon herbes de Provence *or* ¼ teaspoon *each* dried rosemary, thyme, sage and savory
- 4 turnips, peeled and cut into wedges
- 10 ounces fresh brussels sprouts (about 10 medium), trimmed
- 8 ounces baby carrots (about 2 cups)
- 4 ounces pearl onions (about 1 cup), skins removed

1 Heat oil in Dutch oven over medium-high heat. Add roast; cook until browned on all sides.

2 Add broth, garlic and herbes de Provence to Dutch oven; bring to a boil over high heat. Reduce heat to low; cover and simmer 1½ hours.

3 Add turnips, brussels sprouts, carrots and onions to Dutch oven; cover and cook over medium heat 25 to 30 minutes or until vegetables are tender. Remove meat and vegetables; arrange on serving platter. Cover with foil to keep warm.

4 Strain broth; return to Dutch oven. Bring to a boil over medium-high heat; cook until reduced and thickened slightly. Serve immediately with pot roast and vegetables.

Makes 8 servings

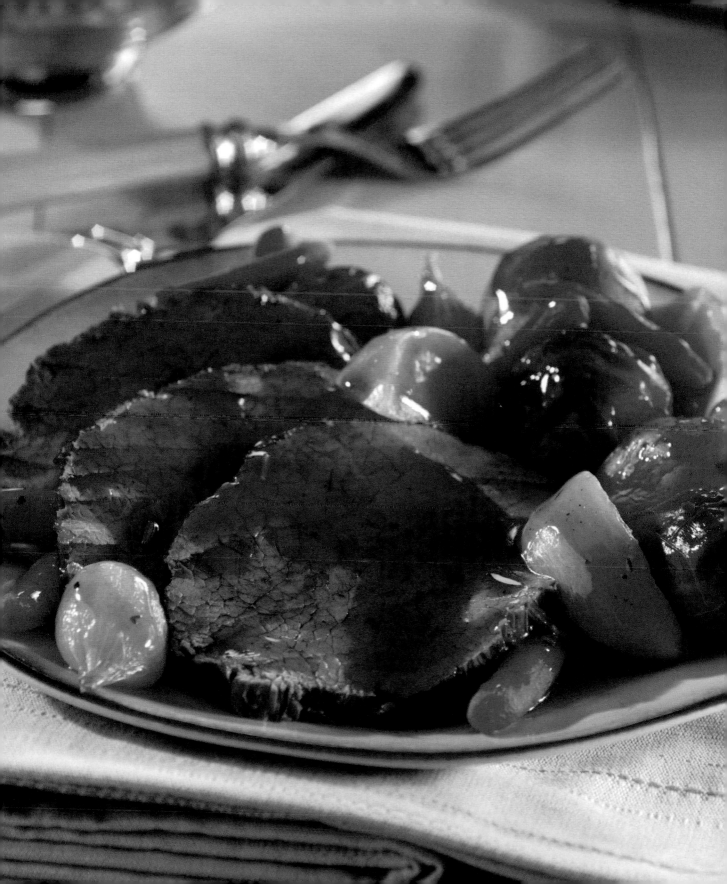

RIB EYE STEAKS WITH CHILI BUTTER

½ cup (1 stick) butter, softened
2 teaspoons chili powder
1 teaspoon minced garlic
1 teaspoon Dijon mustard
⅛ teaspoon ground red pepper or chipotle chile pepper
1 teaspoon black pepper
4 beef rib eye steaks
   Salt

1 Beat butter, chili powder, garlic, mustard and red pepper in medium bowl until smooth. Place mixture on sheet of waxed paper. Roll mixture back and forth into 6-inch log using waxed paper. If butter is too soft, refrigerate up to 30 minutes. Wrap in waxed paper; refrigerate at least 1 hour or up to 2 days.

2 Oil grid. Prepare grill for direct cooking. Rub black pepper over both sides of steaks.

3 Grill steaks, covered, over medium-high heat 8 to 10 minutes or until desired doneness, turning occasionally. Season with salt; serve with slices of Chili Butter.

Makes 4 servings

TIP Butter is a confusing subject in the paleo world. While some argue that no dairy foods of any kind should be consumed, many others believe that organic, grass-fed butter (preferably clarified) does not cause digestive problems and can be part of a healthy diet. You should make the decision that is right for you.

TEXAS MEETS N.Y. STRIP STEAKS

3   tablespoons olive oil, divided
2   medium onions, thinly sliced
4   strip steaks (6 to 8 ounces each)
2   teaspoons minced garlic
2   teaspoons black pepper
    Salt

1 Heat 2 tablespoons oil in medium skillet over medium heat. Add onions; cook and stir 15 to 20 minutes or until soft and golden brown.

2 Meanwhile, prepare grill for direct cooking. Rub steaks with remaining 1 tablespoon oil and garlic. Sprinkle pepper over both sides of steaks.

3 Grill steaks over medium-high heat 10 to 12 minutes until 145°F or until desired doneness, turning twice to obtain cross-hatch grill marks. Season with salt; serve with onions.

Makes 4 servings

TIP New York strip steak is also known as Kansas City steak, shell steak, top loin steak and ambassador steak. It is naturally tender and flavorful (and expensive), often heavily marbled with fat. It comes from the short loin along the back of the cow, an area that gets minimal use—unlike shanks and flanks, there is less muscle so the meat stays tender.

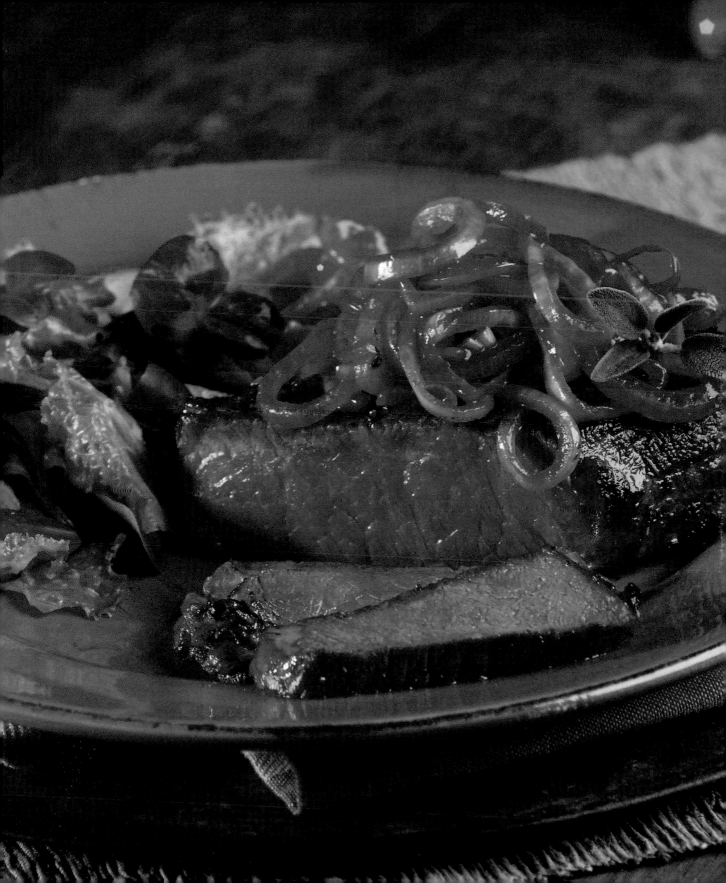

MIDDLE EASTERN BEEF AND EGGPLANT STEW

1 tablespoon olive oil

1 small eggplant, trimmed and cut into 1-inch chunks

2 cups shiitake or cremini mushrooms, quartered

1 can (about 14 ounces) diced tomatoes

½ pound beef top round steak, trimmed and cut into 1-inch pieces

1 medium onion, chopped

1 cup beef broth

1 clove garlic, minced

Grated peel of 1 lemon

½ teaspoon salt

⅓ teaspoon ground cumin

¼ teaspoon red pepper flakes

¼ teaspoon ground cinnamon

⅛ teaspoon black pepper

Slow Cooker Directions

1 Heat oil in large nonstick skillet over medium-high heat. Add eggplant; cook and stir 5 minutes or until lightly browned on all sides. Transfer to 5-quart slow cooker.

2 Stir in remaining ingredients. Cover; cook on LOW 6 hours.

Makes 4 servings

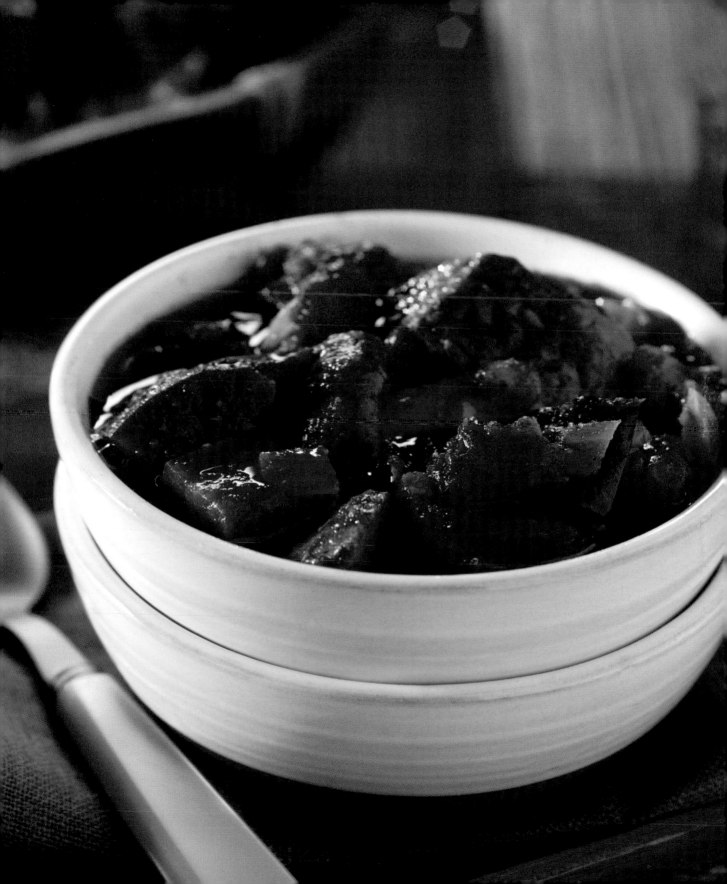

FLANK STEAK AND ROASTED VEGETABLE SALAD

1½ pounds asparagus spears, trimmed and cut into 2-inch lengths
8 ounces baby carrots (about 2 cups)
2 tablespoons olive oil, divided
1 teaspoon salt, divided
1 teaspoon black pepper, divided
1 pound flank steak (1 inch thick)
2 tablespoons plus 1 teaspoon Dijon mustard, divided
1 tablespoon lemon juice
1 tablespoon water
1 teaspoon honey
6 cups mixed salad greens

1 Preheat oven to 400°F. Combine asparagus, carrots, 1 tablespoon oil, ½ teaspoon salt and ¼ teaspoon pepper in shallow roasting pan; toss to coat. Roast 20 minutes or until vegetables are browned and tender, stirring once.

2 Meanwhile, sprinkle steak with ¼ teaspoon salt and ½ teaspoon pepper. Rub both sides of steak with 2 tablespoons mustard. Place steak on rack in baking pan. Roast 10 minutes for medium-rare or until desired doneness, turning once. Let stand 5 minutes.

3 Combine lemon juice, water, honey, remaining 1 tablespoon oil, 1 teaspoon mustard, ¼ teaspoon salt and ¼ teaspoon pepper in large bowl; mix well. Drizzle 1 tablespoon dressing over vegetables in roasting pan; toss to coat.

4 Add greens to dressing in large bowl; toss to coat. Cut steak into thin slices across the grain. Divide greens among four plates; top with steak and vegetables.

Makes 4 servings

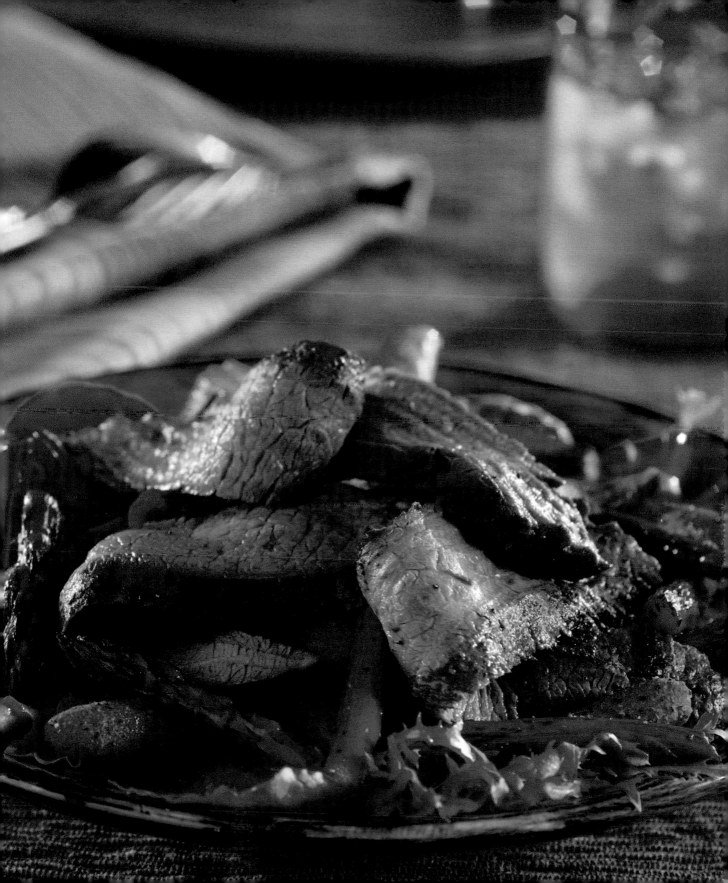

LONDON BROIL WITH MARINATED VEGETABLES

¾ cup olive oil

¾ cup red wine

2 tablespoons finely chopped shallots

2 tablespoons red wine vinegar

2 teaspoons minced garlic

½ teaspoon salt

½ teaspoon dried thyme

½ teaspoon dried oregano

½ teaspoon dried basil

½ teaspoon black pepper

2 pounds top round London broil (1½ inches thick)

1 red onion, cut into ¼-inch-thick slices

1 package (8 ounces) sliced mushrooms

1 red bell pepper, cut into strips

1 zucchini, cut into ¼-inch-thick slices

1 Combine oil, wine, shallots, vinegar, garlic, salt, thyme, oregano, basil and black pepper in medium bowl; mix well.

2 Combine London broil and ¾ cup marinade in large resealable food storage bag. Seal bag; turn to coat. Marinate in refrigerator up to 24 hours, turning bag once or twice.

3 Combine onion, mushrooms, bell pepper, zucchini and remaining marinade in separate large food storage bag. Seal bag; turn to coat. Refrigerate up to 24 hours, turning bag once or twice.

4 Preheat broiler. Remove beef from marinade; discard marinade. Place beef on broiler pan. Broil 4 to 5 inches from heat about 9 minutes per side or until desired doneness. Let stand 10 minutes before cutting into thin slices.

5 Meanwhile, drain vegetables and arrange on broiler pan; discard marinade. Broil 4 to 5 inches from heat about 9 minutes or until edges of vegetables just begin to brown.

Makes 6 servings

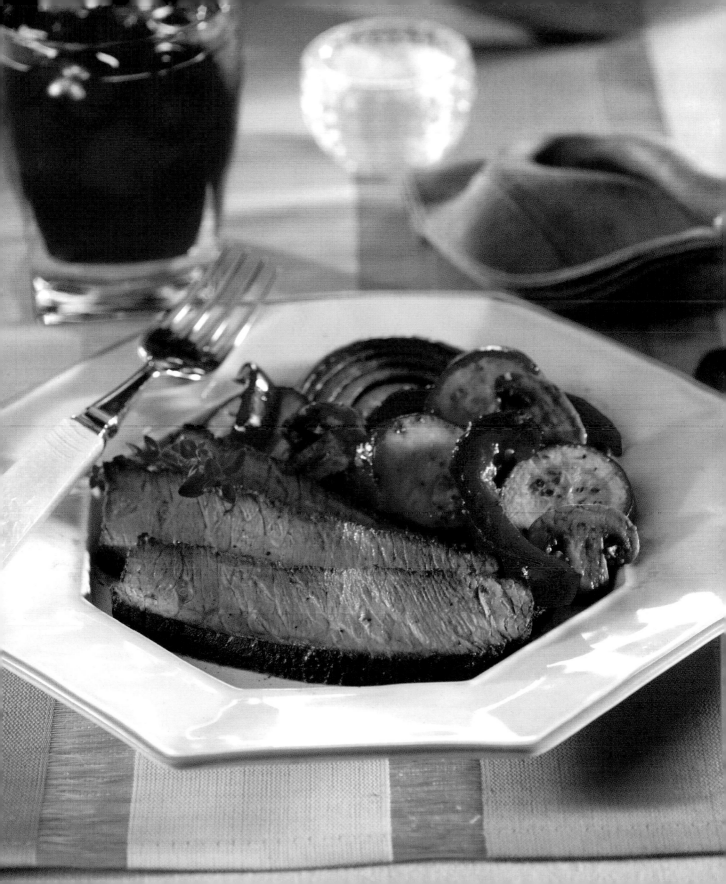

CUBAN-STYLE MARINATED SKIRT STEAK

2 pounds beef skirt steak, cut into 6-inch pieces
2 cups orange juice, divided
½ cup lemon juice
½ cup lime juice
¼ cup olive oil
5 cloves garlic, minced
1 teaspoon dried oregano
½ teaspoon salt
1 large onion, halved and thinly sliced
2 teaspoons grated orange peel

1 Place steaks in large resealable food storage bag. Combine 1 cup orange juice, lemon juice, lime juice, oil, garlic, oregano and salt in medium bowl; mix well. Set aside ½ cup marinade for serving. Pour remaining mixture over steaks. Seal bag; turn to coat. Marinate in refrigerator 30 minutes.

2 Combine remaining 1 cup orange juice, onion and orange peel in small bowl; set aside.

3 Prepare grill for direct cooking. Remove steaks from marinade; discard marinade. Grill steaks, covered, over high heat 6 to 10 minutes or until desired doneness, turning once. Tent with foil; let stand 5 minutes.

4 Drain onion; discard liquid. Cut steaks into thin slices against the grain. Transfer to serving platter; sprinkle with onion and reserved ½ cup marinade.

Makes 6 servings

TIP: Traditionally used for fajitas, skirt steaks are long, narrow, thin cuts of meat with a distinct visible grain. They are easier to grill if cut into smaller portions. For maximum tenderness, cut cooked steaks against the grain into thin slices. Tilt the knife diagonally when cutting to ensure the largest surface area possible for each slice.

CINNAMON-SPIKED BEEF AND TOMATO STEW

- 1 pound boneless beef sirloin tri-tip roast, trimmed*
- 1 tablespoon olive oil
- 1 medium sweet onion, halved and cut into ½-inch thick slices
- 1 can (28 ounces) crushed tomatoes in purée
- 1 cup beef broth
- 1 tablespoon cider vinegar
- 2 teaspoons grated orange peel
- 1 teaspoon ground cinnamon
- ½ teaspoon salt
- ½ teaspoon ground ginger
- 2 sweet potatoes, cut into 1-inch pieces (about 4 cups)
- 3 carrots, cut into 1-inch pieces
- 2 cooking apples, peeled and cut into 1-inch pieces
- 3 tablespoons chopped fresh parsley

Substitute chuck roast or beef round steak, if desired.

1 Cut beef into 1-inch pieces. Heat oil in large saucepan or Dutch oven over medium heat. Add half of beef; cook and stir until browned. Remove to plate. Repeat with remaining beef. Return all beef to saucepan.

2 Add onion to saucepan; cook about 4 minutes or until tender, stirring occasionally. Stir in tomatoes, broth, vinegar, orange peel, cinnamon, salt and ginger; bring to a boil. Reduce heat to medium-low; simmer, uncovered, 10 minutes.

3 Stir in sweet potatoes, carrots and apples; bring to a boil over high heat. Reduce heat to low; cover and simmer about 1 hour or until vegetables are tender. Garnish with parsley.

Makes 6 servings

FLANK STEAK WITH ITALIAN SALSA

- 2 tablespoons olive oil
- 2 teaspoons balsamic vinegar
- 1 lean flank steak (1½ pounds)
- 1 tablespoon minced garlic
- ¾ teaspoon salt, divided
- ¾ teaspoon black pepper, divided
- 1 cup diced plum tomatoes
- ⅓ cup chopped pitted kalamata olives
- 2 tablespoons chopped fresh basil

1 Whisk oil and vinegar in medium bowl until well blended. Place steak in shallow dish; spread garlic over both sides of steak. Sprinkle with ½ teaspoon salt and ½ teaspoon pepper; drizzle with 2 tablespoons oil mixture. (Reserve remaining mixture for salsa.) Cover and marinate steak in refrigerator at least 20 minutes or up to 2 hours.

2 Prepare grill for direct cooking or preheat broiler. Add tomatoes, olives, basil, remaining ¼ teaspoon salt and ¼ teaspoon pepper to oil mixture remaining in bowl; mix well.

3 Remove steak from marinade. (Let garlic remain on steak.) Grill steak over medium-high heat 5 to 6 minutes per side for medium-rare or until desired doneness. Remove to cutting board. Tent steak with foil; let stand 5 minutes.

4 Cut steak diagonally into thin slices across the grain. Serve with salsa.

Makes 4 servings

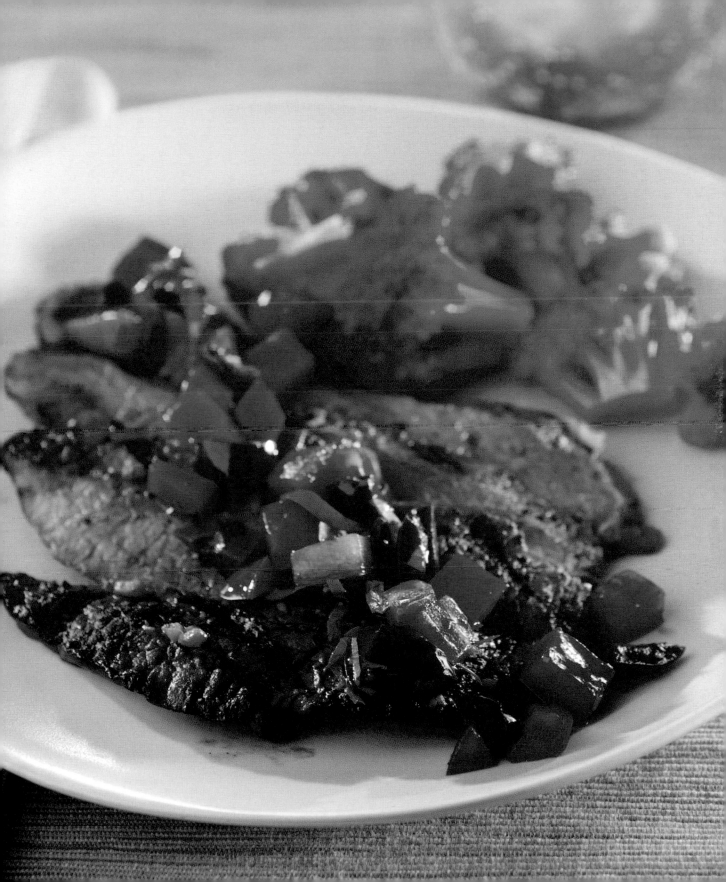

BEEF AND PEPPER KABOBS

. . . .

    8 ounces sirloin steak
    2 teaspoons coconut aminos*
    2 teaspoons red wine vinegar
 1½ teaspoons Dijon mustard
    1 teaspoon olive oil
    1 clove garlic, minced
  ⅛ teaspoon black pepper
    2 bell peppers (any color or a combination)
    4 green onions, trimmed

Coconut aminos is a dark, salty soy-free sauce containing 17 amino acids. It is made from the sap of the coconut tree which is dried and blended with sea salt. It does not have a pronounced coconut flavor and is often used as a substitute for soy sauce in paleo recipes. Coconut aminos can be found in health food and vitamin stores, some grocery stores or online.

1 Cut steak into 16 (¼-inch-thick) strips; place in glass bowl. Whisk coconut aminos, vinegar, mustard, oil, garlic and black pepper in medium bowl until well blended. Add half of marinade to beef; toss to coat. Cover and marinate in refrigerator 2 to 3 hours, stirring occasionally. Place remaining marinade in small bowl; cover and refrigerate.

2 Oil grid. Prepare grill for direct cooking. Cut each bell pepper into 12 pieces. Thread six bell pepper pieces onto each of four metal skewers. Grill bell peppers 5 to 7 minutes per side or until well browned and tender.

3 Add green onions to grid; grill 3 to 5 minutes or until well browned on both sides. Brush bell peppers and green onions lightly with reserved marinade once during grilling.

4 Thread four beef strips onto each of four skewers. Grill 2 minutes per side, lightly basting once per side with marinade.

5 To serve, place one beef skewer and one bell pepper skewer on each of four plates. Remove beef and bell peppers from skewers. Chop green onions; sprinkle over each serving.

Makes 4 servings

. . . .

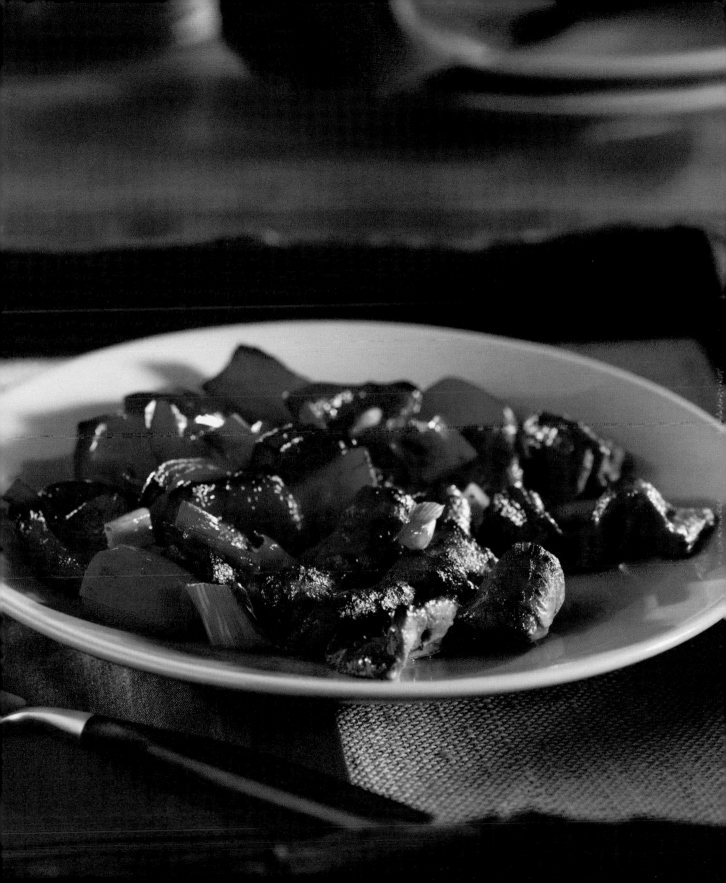

SKIRT STEAK WITH RED PEPPER CHIMICHURRI

1 **cup diced roasted red bell pepper**
2 **tablespoons olive oil, divided**
1 **shallot, minced**
1 **tablespoon capers**
1 **tablespoon white wine vinegar**
1 **clove garlic, minced**
1 **pound skirt steak, trimmed**
1 **clove garlic, peeled and cut in half**
¼ **teaspoon salt**
½ **teaspoon black pepper, divided**

1 For chimichurri, combine roasted pepper, 1½ tablespoons oil, shallot, capers, vinegar, minced garlic and ¼ teaspoon black pepper in medium bowl; mix well.

2 Preheat broiler. Brush broiler rack with remaining ½ tablespoon oil.

3 Rub steak on both sides with garlic clove. Season with salt and remaining ¼ teaspoon black pepper. Place steak on broiler rack; broil 4 inches from heat 4 to 5 minutes per side or until desired doneness. Let stand 5 minutes.

4 Cut steak into thin slices against the grain; arrange on platter. Top with chimichurri or serve sauce separately.

Makes 4 servings

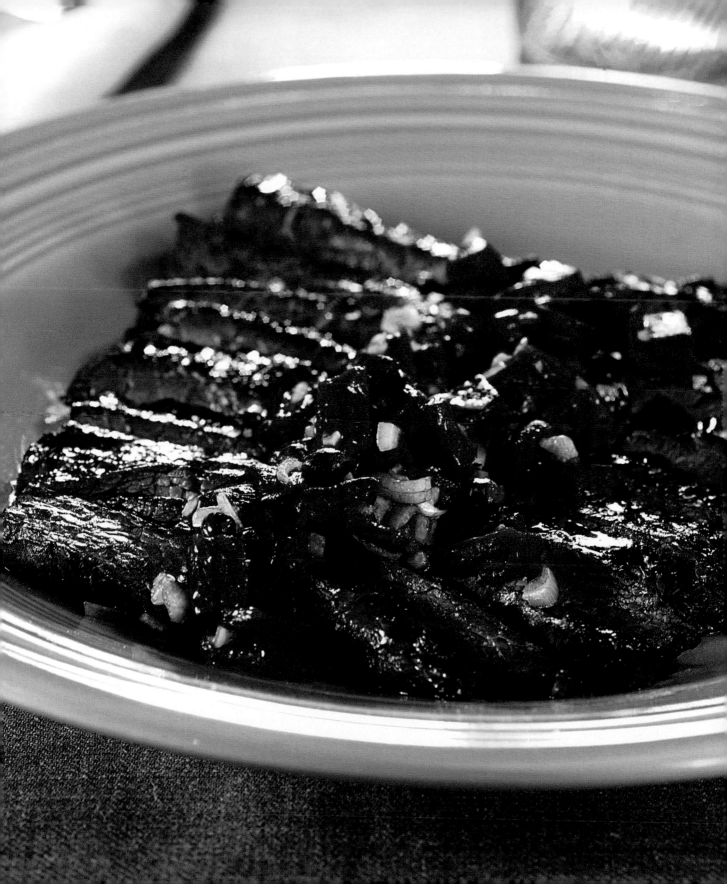

SWISS STEAK STEW

2 to 3 boneless beef top sirloin steaks (about 4 pounds)

2 cans (about 14 ounces each) diced tomatoes

2 green bell peppers, cut into ½-inch strips

2 onions, chopped

1 tablespoon seasoned salt blend*

1 teaspoon black pepper

Many seasoned salts contain processed ingredients and/or fillers. Check ingredient labels and look for blends that contain only all-natural sea salt, herbs and spices.

Slow Cooker Directions

Cut each steak into 3 to 4 pieces; place in slow cooker. Add tomatoes, bell peppers and onions. Sprinkle with seasoned salt and black pepper. Cover; cook on LOW 8 hours or until beef is tender.

Makes 10 servings

STEAK AL FORNO

4 cloves garlic, minced

1 tablespoon olive oil

1 tablespoon coarse salt

1 teaspoon black pepper

2 porterhouse or T-bone steaks (1 to 1¼ inches thick)

1 Prepare grill for direct cooking. Combine garlic, oil, salt and pepper in small bowl; press into both sides of steaks. Let stand 15 minutes.

2 Grill steaks, covered, over medium-high heat 7 to 10 minutes per side for medium-rare (145°F) or until desired doneness. Transfer to cutting board; tent with foil. Let stand 5 minutes.

3 To serve, cut meat away from each side of bone. Cut boneless pieces into slices. Serve immediately.

Makes 2 to 3 servings

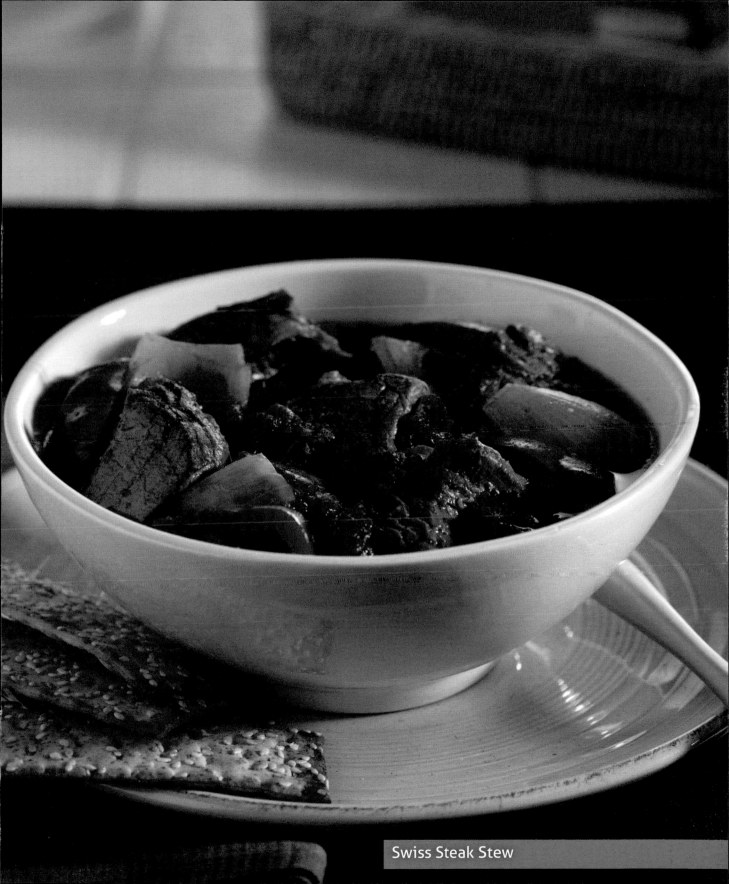

Swiss Steak Stew

PORK

BALSAMIC GRILLED PORK CHOPS

- 2 **tablespoons balsamic vinegar**
- 2 **tablespoons coconut aminos***
- 1 **teaspoon Dijon mustard**
- 1 **teaspoon honey**
- ⅛ **teaspoon red pepper flakes**
- 2 **boneless pork chops, trimmed (about 4 ounces each)**
- 2 **teaspoons olive oil**

*Coconut aminos is a dark, salty soy-free sauce containing 17 amino acids. It is made from the sap of the coconut tree which is dried and blended with sea salt. It does not have a pronounced coconut flavor and is often used as a substitute for soy sauce in paleo recipes. Coconut aminos can be found in health food and vitamin stores, some grocery stores or online.

1 Combine vinegar, coconut aminos, mustard, honey and red pepper flakes in small bowl; mix well. Reserve 1 tablespoon marinade; refrigerate until ready to serve.

2 Place pork in large resealable food storage bag. Pour remaining marinade over pork. Seal bag; turn to coat. Marinate in refrigerator 2 hours or up to 24 hours.

3 Bursh grill pan with oil; heat over medium-high heat. Remove pork from marinade; discard marinade. Cook pork 4 minutes per side or until barely pink in center. Drizzle with reserved 1 tablespoon marinade.

Makes 2 servings

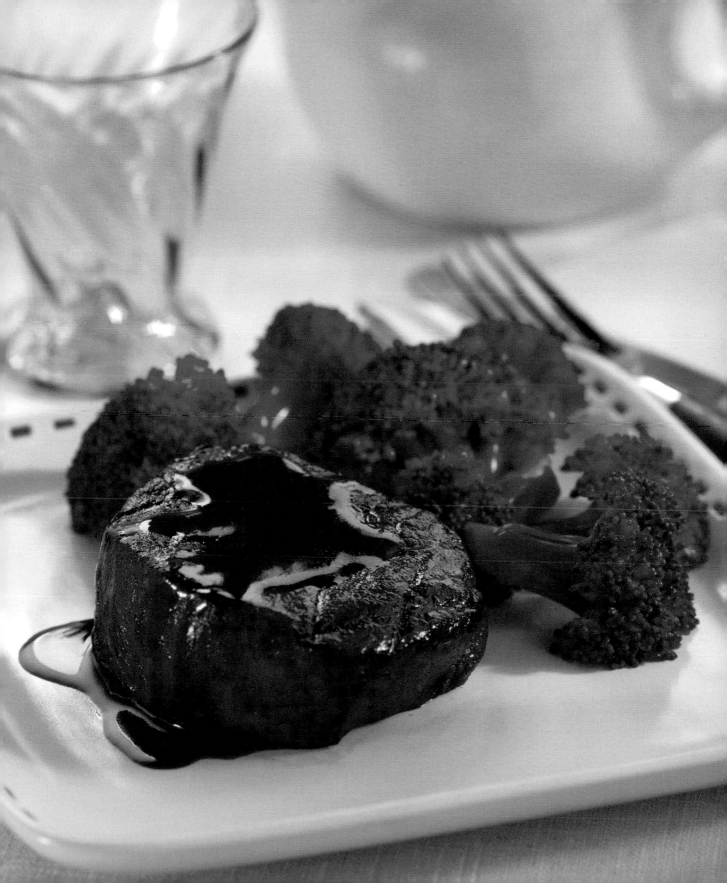

PORK AND CABBAGE SOUP

- 8 ounces pork loin, cut into ½-inch cubes
- 1 medium onion, chopped
- 2 slices bacon, finely chopped
- 2 cups beef broth
- 2 cup chicken broth
- 1 can (about 28 ounces) whole tomatoes, drained and coarsely chopped
- 2 medium carrots, sliced
- 1 bay leaf
- 1 teaspoon salt
- ¾ teaspoon dried marjoram
- ⅛ teaspoon black pepper
- ¼ medium cabbage, chopped
- 2 tablespoons chopped fresh parsley

1 Heat large saucepan or Dutch oven over medium heat. Add pork, onion and bacon; cook and stir until pork is no longer pink and onion is slightly tender. Drain fat.

2 Stir in beef broth, chicken broth, tomatoes, carrots, bay leaf, salt, marjoram and pepper; bring to a boil over high heat. Reduce heat to medium-low; simmer, uncovered, about 30 minutes. Remove and discard bay leaf. Skim off fat.

3 Add cabbage; bring to a boil over high heat. Reduce heat to medium-low; simmer, uncovered, about 15 minutes or until cabbage is tender. Stir in parsley.

Makes 6 servings

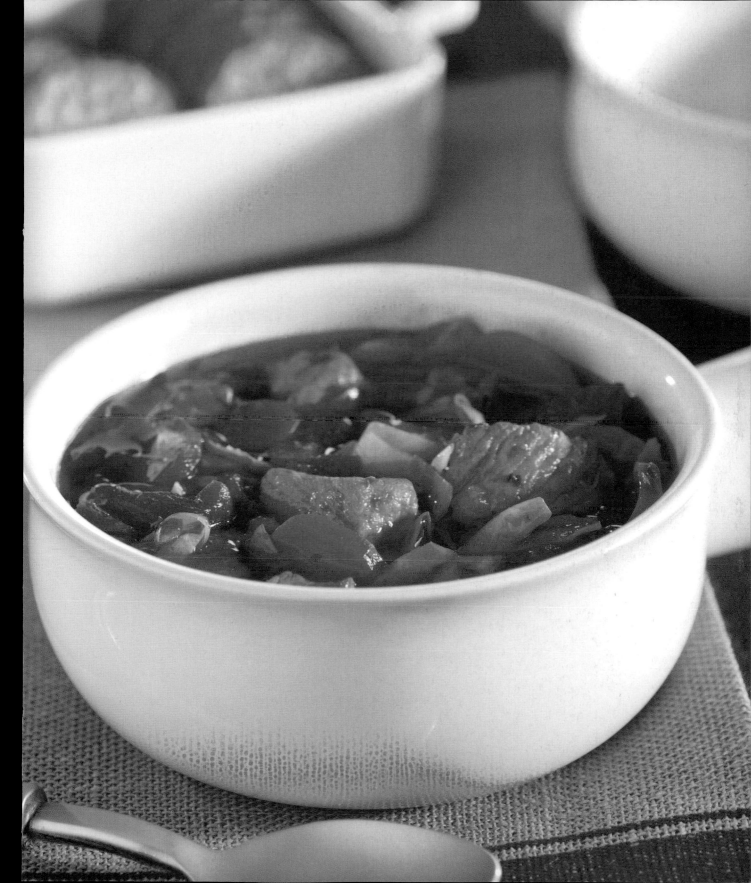

QUICK AND EASY PORK CHOPS WITH APPLES

- 1 **tablespoon olive oil**
- 4 **bone-in pork chops, cut ¾-inch thick**
  Salt and black pepper
- 2 **to 3 apples, cored and sliced**
- 1½ **cups dry white wine**

1 Heat oil in large skillet over medium heat. Brown pork on both sides; season with salt and pepper.

2 Add apples and wine, stirring to scrape up browned bits from bottom of skillet. Reduce heat to medium-low; cover and cook 20 to 25 minutes or until barely pink in center. Remove pork to platter; keep warm.

3 Bring apples and wine to a boil over medium-high heat; cook 5 minutes or until liquid is reduced by half. Serve with pork.

Makes 4 servings

VARIATION: Season chops with a mixture of ¼ teaspoon *each* dried thyme, garlic salt and black pepper before browning.

NOTE: If using boneless pork loin chops, cook 10 to 15 minutes.

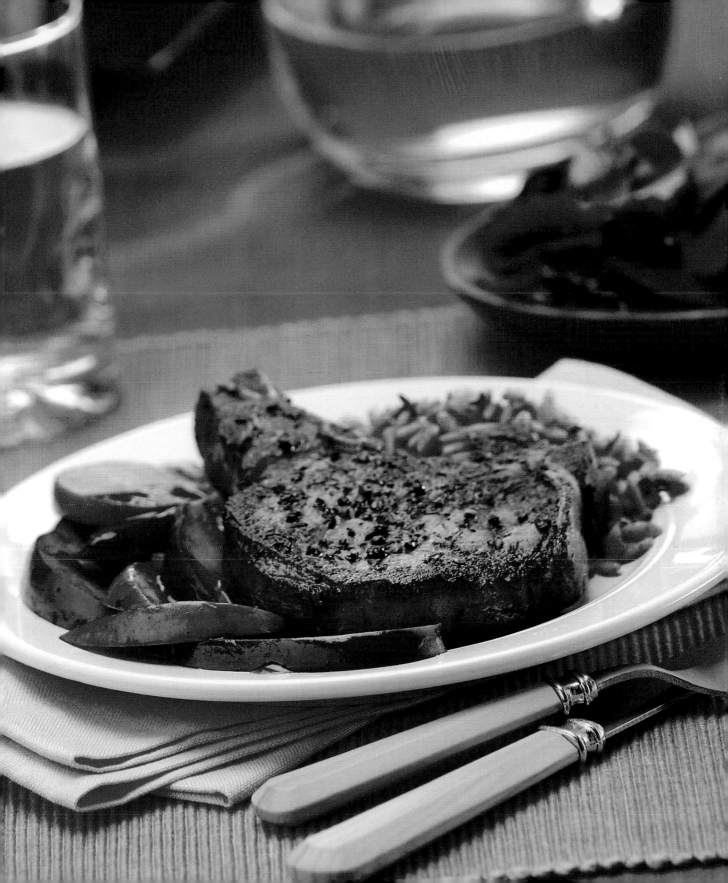

PORK ROAST WITH DIJON TARRAGON GLAZE

⅓ cup chicken or vegetable broth
2 tablespoons lemon juice
2 tablespoons Dijon mustard
1 teaspoon minced fresh tarragon
1½ to 2 pounds boneless pork loin, visible fat removed
1 teaspoon ground paprika
½ teaspoon black pepper

Slow Cooker Directions

1 Combine broth, lemon juice, mustard and tarragon in small bowl; mix well. Sprinkle pork with paprika and pepper; place in slow cooker. Spoon mustard mixture evenly over pork. Cover; cook on LOW 6 to 8 hours or on HIGH 3 to 4 hours.

2 Remove pork from slow cooker; let stand 15 minutes before slicing.

Make 4 to 6 servings

MAPLE-MUSTARD PORK CHOPS

2 tablespoons maple syrup, divided
2 tablespoons olive oil, divided
2 teaspoons whole grain mustard
2 center-cut pork loin chops (about 6 ounces each)
⅓ cup water

1 Preheat oven to 375°F. Combine maple syrup, 1 tablespoon oil and mustard in small bowl; mix well. Brush over both sides of pork.

2 Heat remaining 1 tablespoon oil in medium ovenproof skillet over medium-high heat. Add pork; cook until browned on both sides. Add water; cover and bake 20 to 30 minutes or until pork is barely pink in center.

Makes 2 servings

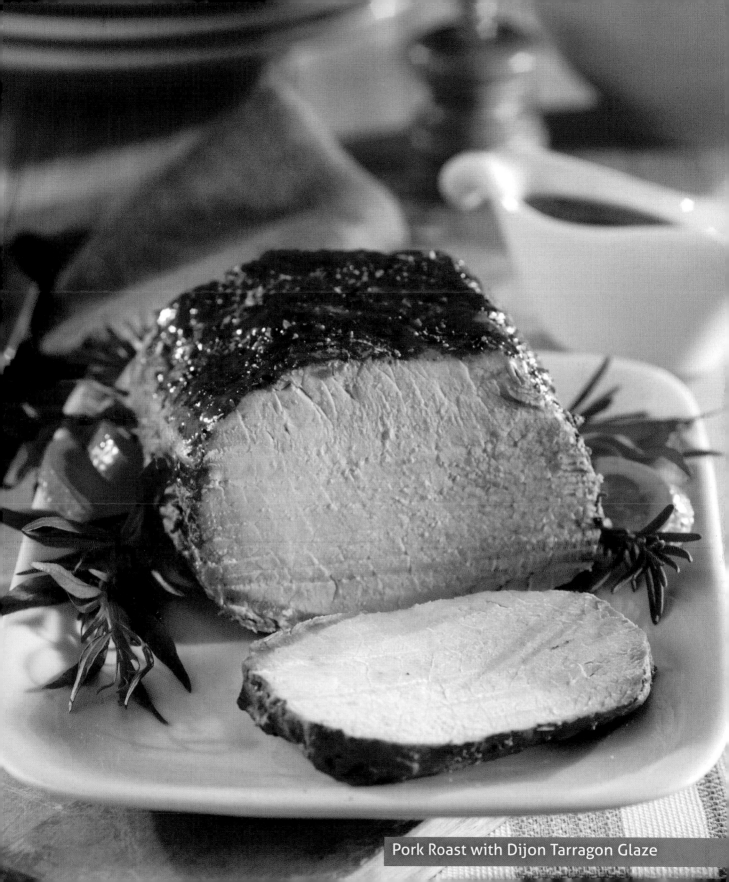

Pork Roast with Dijon Tarragon Glaze

PORK CHOPS WITH VINEGAR PEPPERS

          4 pork rib chops (about 1 inch thick)
        ½ teaspoon salt
        ¼ teaspoon black pepper
          2 tablespoons olive oil
     1½ cups sliced seeded hot cherry peppers (½-inch slices)
          2 cloves garlic, minced
        ¼ cup liquid from cherry pepper jar
        ¼ cup water
          1 sprig fresh rosemary
             Chopped fresh Italian parsley (optional)

1 Pat pork chops dry with paper towels. Season both sides of pork with salt and pepper.

2 Heat oil in large saucepan over medium-high heat. Add pork; cook about 5 minutes per side or until browned. Remove from skillet; keep warm.

3 Add cherry peppers and garlic to skillet; cook and stir 2 minutes over medium heat, scraping up browned bits from bottom of pan. Stir in cherry pepper liquid, water and rosemary.

4 Return pork chops along with any accumulated juices to skillet; cover and cook about 6 minutes or until pork is barely pink in center. Sprinkle with parsley, if desired.

Makes 4 servings

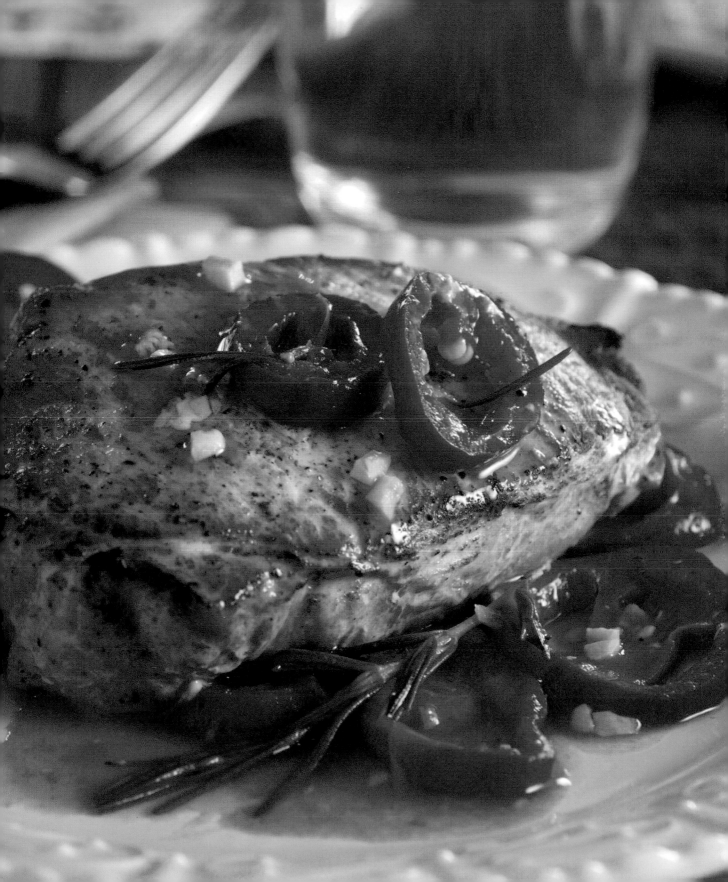

SPICY PORK AND VEGETABLE STEW

- 1 tablespoon olive oil
- 1½ pounds boneless pork loin, trimmed and cut into ½-inch cubes
- 1 cup chopped onion
- 2 red bell peppers, cut into ½-inch pieces
- 1 package (8 ounces) sliced mushrooms
- 1 medium acorn squash, peeled and cut into ½-inch cubes
- 1 can (about 14 ounces) diced tomatoes
- 1¾ cups chicken broth
- ½ teaspoon dried thyme
- ½ teaspoon red pepper flakes
- ½ teaspoon black pepper
  Fresh oregano (optional)

1 Heat oil in large saucepan or Dutch oven over medium-high heat. Add half of pork; cook about 5 minutes or until browned, stirring occasionally. Remove to plate. Repeat with remaining pork.

2 Add onion, bell peppers and mushrooms to saucepan. Stir in pork, squash, tomatoes, broth, thyme, red pepper flakes and black pepper; bring to a boil over high heat. Reduce heat to medium-low; cover and simmer 1 hour or until pork is tender. Garnish with oregano.

Makes 6 to 8 servings

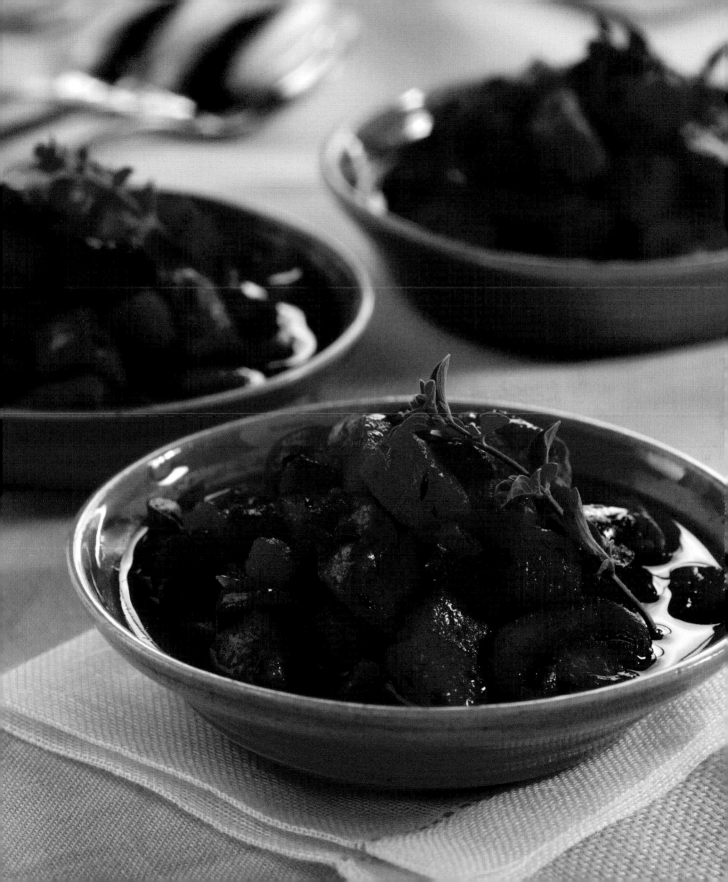

MAPLE AND SAGE PORK CHOPS

- 2 tablespoons finely chopped fresh sage, plus additional for garnish
- 1 tablespoon olive oil
- ½ teaspoon salt
- 4 boneless pork chops (about 4 ounces each)
- 1 tablespoon maple syrup

1 Preheat broiler. Combine 2 tablespoons sage, oil and salt in small bowl; mix well. Rub over both sides of pork. Place on rimmed baking sheet.

2 Broil pork chops 4 minutes. Turn pork and brush evenly with syrup. Broil 4 minutes or until pork is browned and barely pink in center. Garnish with additional sage.

Makes 4 servings

PORK IN CHILE SAUCE

- 1 large tomato, chopped
- 1 cup tomato purée
- 1 small poblano pepper, seeded and chopped
- 1 large shallot *or* ½ small onion, chopped
- 1 clove garlic, minced
- ¼ teaspoon dried oregano
- ⅛ teaspoon chipotle chili powder or regular chili powder
- ⅛ teaspoon black pepper
- 1 boneless pork chop (about 6 ounces), cut into 1-inch pieces
- ¼ teaspoon salt

Slow Cooker Directions

Combine tomato, tomato purée, poblano, shallot, garlic, oregano, chili powder and black pepper in slow cooker; mix well. Add pork. Cover; cook on LOW 5 to 6 hours. Stir in salt.

Makes 2 servings

NOTE: This recipe works best in a small (1½-quart) slow cooker.

Maple and Sage Pork Chops

ROASTED PORK TENDERLOIN WITH FRESH PLUM SALSA

Fresh Plum Salsa (recipe follows)
1 **pound pork tenderloin, trimmed**
¼ **cup coconut aminos**
2 **tablespoons lime juice**
2 **teaspoons dark sesame oil**
2 **cloves garlic, minced**
1½ **tablespoons honey**

1 Prepare Fresh Plum Salsa.

2 Place pork in large resealable food storage bag. Combine coconut aminos, lime juice, oil and garlic in small bowl; mix well. Pour over pork. Seal bag; turn to coat. Marinate in refrigerator 8 hours or overnight, turning occasionally.

3 Preheat oven to 375°F. Remove pork from marinade, reserving 2 tablespoons marinade in small saucepan. Add honey to saucepan; bring to a boil over medium-high heat. Boil 1 minute, stirring once.

4 To ensure even cooking, tuck narrow end of pork under roast to form even thickness. Tie with cotton string. Place pork on rack in shallow roasting pan; brush with honey mixture.

5 Roast 15 minutes; brush with remaining honey mixture. Roast 10 minutes or until 145°F. Transfer pork to cutting board. Tent with foil; let stand 10 minutes.

6 Remove string from pork. Cut into thin slices; serve with salsa.

Makes 4 servings

FRESH PLUM SALSA

2 **cups coarsely chopped red plums (about 3)**
2 **tablespoons chopped green onion**
1 **tablespoon honey**
1 **tablespoon chopped fresh cilantro**
2 **teaspoons lime juice**
Dash ground red pepper

Combine all ingredients in medium bowl; mix well. Cover and refrigerate at least 2 hours.

Makes 1 cup

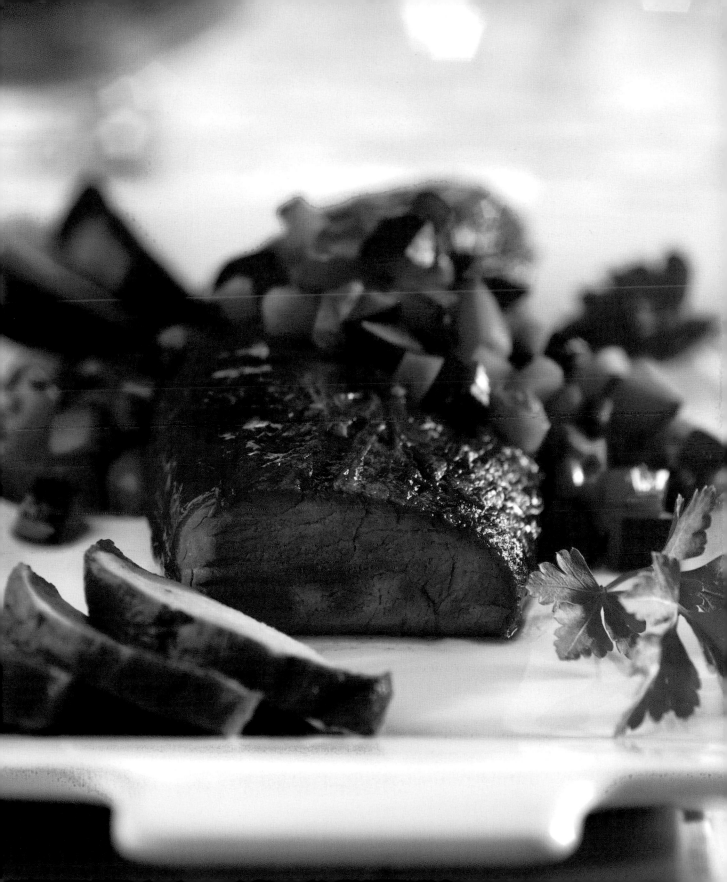

CUBAN GARLIC AND LIME PORK CHOPS

- 4 boneless pork top loin chops, ¾ inch thick (about 6 ounces each)
- 2 tablespoons olive oil
- 2 tablespoons lime juice
- 2 tablespoons orange juice
- 2 teaspoons minced garlic
- ½ teaspoon salt, divided
- ½ teaspoon red pepper flakes
- 2 small seedless oranges, peeled and chopped
- 1 medium cucumber, peeled, seeded and chopped
- 2 tablespoons chopped onion
- 2 tablespoons chopped fresh cilantro

1 Place pork in large resealable food storage bag. Add oil, lime juice, orange juice, garlic, ¼ teaspoon salt and red pepper flakes. Seal bag; turn to coat. Marinate in refrigerator up to 24 hours.

2 Combine oranges, cucumber, onion and cilantro in medium bowl; toss gently. Cover and refrigerate salsa at least 1 hour or overnight. Add remaining ¼ teaspoon salt just before serving.

3 Prepare grill for direct cooking or preheat broiler. Remove pork from marinade; discard marinade. Grill or broil pork 6 to 8 minutes per side or until pork is no longer pink in center. Serve with salsa.

Makes 4 servings

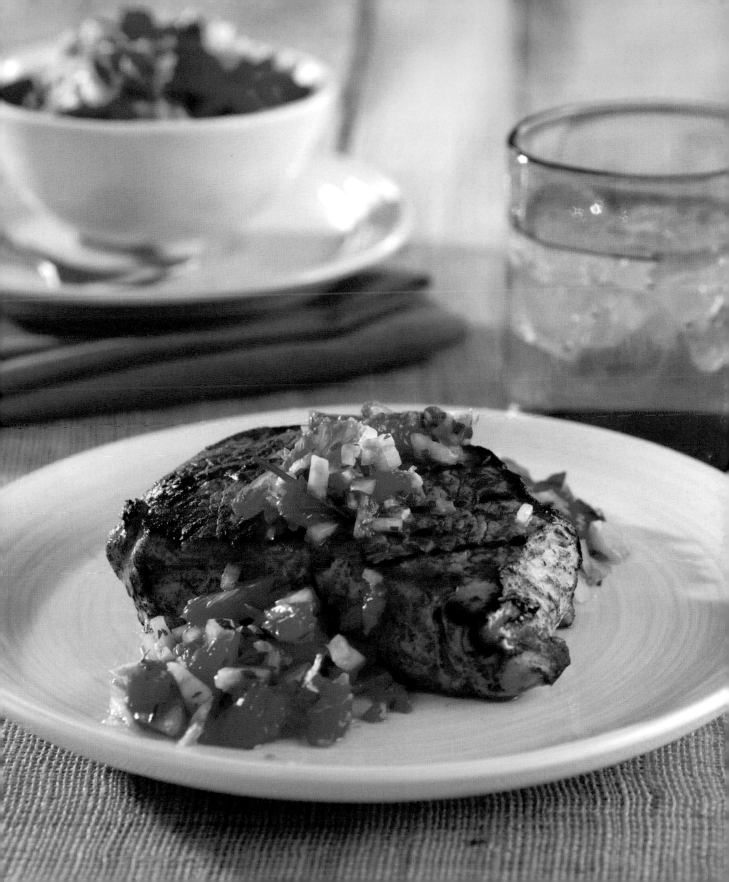

CIDER PORK AND ONIONS

- 2 to 3 tablespoons vegetable oil
- 4 to 4½ pounds bone-in pork shoulder roast (pork butt), trimmed
- 4 to 5 medium onions, sliced (about 4 cups)
- 1 teaspoon salt, divided
- 4 cloves garlic, minced
- 3 sprigs fresh rosemary
- ½ teaspoon black pepper
- 2 to 3 cups apple cider

1 Preheat oven to 325°F. Heat 2 tablespoons oil in Dutch oven over medium-high heat. Add pork; brown on all sides. Remove to plate.

2 Add onions and ½ teaspoon salt to Dutch oven; cook and stir 10 minutes or until translucent, adding additional oil as needed to prevent scorching. Add garlic; cook and stir 1 minute. Add pork and rosemary; sprinkle with remaining ½ teaspoon salt and pepper. Add cider to come about halfway up sides of pork.

3 Cover and bake 2 to 2½ hours or until very tender. (Meat should be almost falling off bones.) Remove to large platter; keep warm.

4 Remove rosemary sprigs from Dutch oven. Boil liquid in Dutch oven over medium-high heat about 20 minutes or until reduced by half; skim fat. Season with additional salt and pepper, if desired. Slice pork; serve with sauce.

Makes 8 servings

CARNITAS

· · · · · · · ·

   2 to 2½ pounds pork shoulder roast (pork butt), trimmed
   2 bay leaves
   2 cloves garlic, minced
   1 teaspoon chili powder
  ¾ teaspoon salt
  ½ teaspoon black pepper
  ½ teaspoon dried oregano
  ½ teaspoon ground cumin
  ½ cup water
     Guacamole (recipe follows) or salsa (optional)

1 Preheat oven to 350°F. Cut pork into 1-inch cubes.

2 Combine bay leaves, garlic, chili powder, salt, pepper, oregano and cumin in small bowl; stir in water until well blended. Place pork in shallow roasting pan. Pour spice mixture over pork; turn to coat. Cover with foil.

3 Bake 45 minutes. Remove foil; bake 45 to 60 minutes or until most of liquid has evaporated and pork begins to brown. Remove and discard bay leaves. Pull pork into large shreds or chunks. Meanwhile, prepare Guacamole, if desired. Serve with pork.

Makes 10 to 12 servings

· · · · · · · · · ·

GUACAMOLE

· · · · · · · ·

   2 large avocados, peeled and pitted
  ¼ cup finely chopped tomato
   2 tablespoons lime juice or lemon juice
   2 tablespoons grated onion with juice
  ½ teaspoon salt
  ¼ teaspoon hot pepper sauce
     Black pepper

Place avocados in medium bowl; mash coarsely with fork. Stir in tomato, lime juice, onion, salt and hot pepper sauce; mix well. Season with black pepper. Serve immediately or cover and refrigerate up to 2 hours.

Makes 2 cups

· · · · · ·

ZESTY SKILLET PORK CHOPS

- 1 teaspoon chili powder
- ½ teaspoon salt, divided
- 4 boneless pork chops (about 6 ounces each)
- 2 cups diced tomatoes
- 1 cup chopped green, red or yellow bell pepper
- ¾ cup thinly sliced celery
- ½ cup chopped onion
- 1 tablespoon hot pepper sauce
- 1 teaspoon dried thyme leaves
- 1 tablespoon olive oil
- 2 tablespoons finely chopped parsley

1 Rub chili powder and ¼ teaspoon salt evenly over one side of pork chops.

2 Combine tomatoes, bell pepper, celery, onion, hot pepper sauce and thyme in medium bowl; mix well.

3 Heat oil in large skillet over medium-high heat. Add pork, seasoned side down; cook 1 minute. Turn pork and top with tomato mixture; bring to a boil.

4 Reduce heat to low; cover and simmer 25 minutes or until pork is tender and sauce has thickened.

5 Remove pork to serving plates; keep warm. Bring sauce to a boil over high heat; cook 2 minutes or until most of liquid has evaporated. Remove from heat; stir in parsley and remaining ¼ teaspoon salt. Serve over pork.

Makes 4 servings

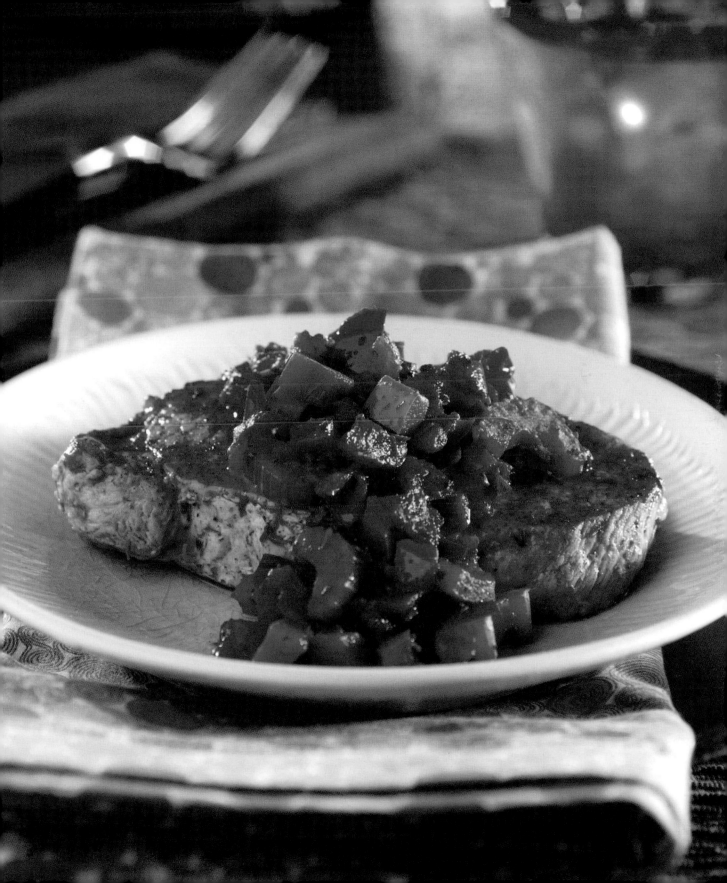

PORK CURRY OVER CAULIFLOWER COUSCOUS

- 3 tablespoons olive oil, divided
- 2 tablespoons mild curry powder
- 2 teaspoons minced garlic
- 1½ pounds boneless pork (shoulder, loin or chops), cubed
- 1 red or green bell pepper, diced
- 1 tablespoon cider vinegar
- ½ teaspoon salt
- 2 cups water
- 1 large head cauliflower

1 Heat 2 tablespoons oil in large saucepan over medium heat. Add curry powder and garlic; cook and stir 1 to 2 minutes or until garlic is golden.

2 Add pork; cook and stir 5 to 7 minutes or until pork is barely pink in center. Add bell pepper and vinegar; cook and stir 3 minutes or until bell pepper is tender. Sprinkle with salt.

3 Add water; bring to a boil. Reduce heat to low; simmer 30 to 45 minutes or until liquid is reduced and pork is tender, stirring occasionally and adding additional water as needed.

4 Meanwhile, trim and core cauliflower; cut into 2-inch pieces. Place in food processor; pulse until cauliflower is in small uniform pieces about the size of cooked couscous. *Do not purée.*

5 Heat remaining 1 tablespoon oil in large skillet over medium heat. Add cauliflower; cook and stir 5 minutes or until crisp-tender. *Do not overcook.* Serve pork over cauliflower.

Makes 6 servings

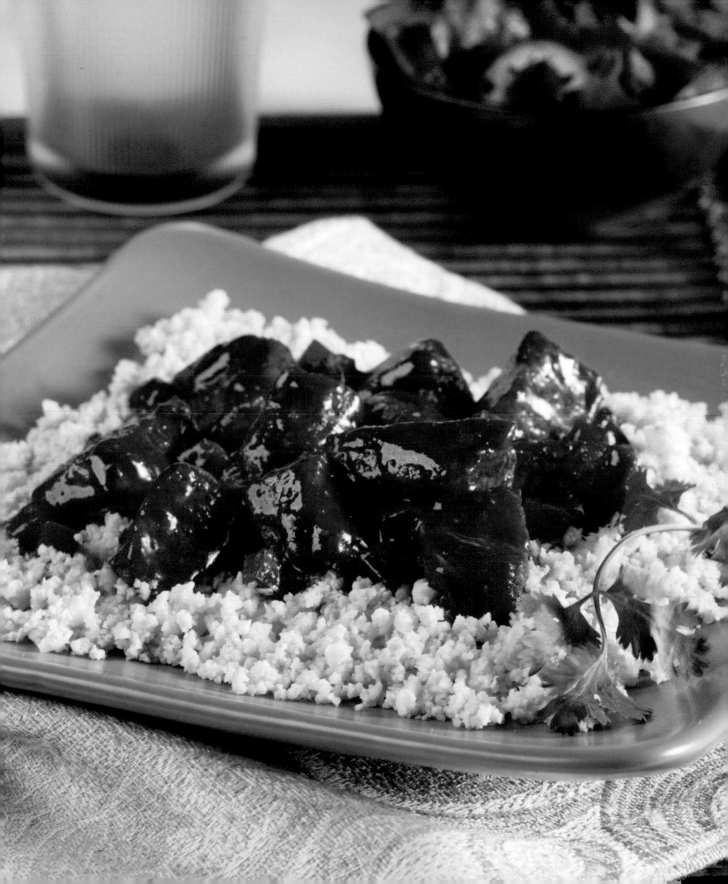

SPICED PORK TENDERLOIN AND APPLES

½ teaspoon salt
½ teaspoon ground cinnamon
½ teaspoon ground cumin
½ teaspoon black pepper
⅛ teaspoon ground allspice
1 pound pork tenderloin
1 tablespoon olive oil
2 medium Fuji or Gala apples, sliced
¼ cup raisins
¼ cup water

1 Preheat oven to 425°F. Line baking sheet with foil.

2 Combine salt, cinnamon, cumin, pepper and allspice in small bowl; mix well. Sprinkle mixture over pork, pressing to adhere.

3 Heat oil in large skillet over medium-high heat. Add pork; cook until browned on all sides, turning frequently. Remove to prepared baking sheet.

4 Bake 18 minutes or until barely pink in center. Remove to cutting board; let stand 5 minutes.

5 Meanwhile, combine apples, raisins and water in same skillet; cook and stir over medium-high heat 3 minutes or until apples begin to brown. Cover and let stand until ready to serve. Cut pork into thin slices; serve with apple mixture.

Makes 4 servings

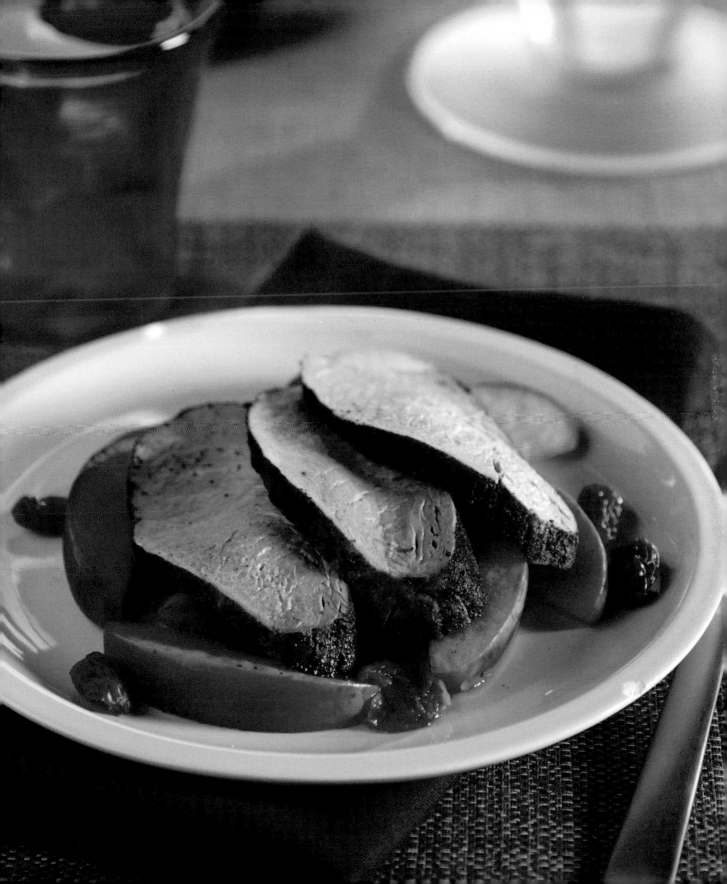

SAGE-ROASTED PORK WITH RUTABAGA

- 1 bunch fresh sage
- 4 cloves garlic, minced (2 tablespoons)
- 1½ teaspoons coarse salt, divided
- 1 teaspoon coarsely ground black pepper, divided
- 5 tablespoons extra virgin olive oil, divided
- 1 boneless pork loin roast (2 to 2½ pounds)
- 2 medium or 1 large rutabaga (1 to 1½ pounds)
- 4 carrots, cut into 1½-inch pieces

1 Chop enough sage to measure 2 tablespoons; reserve remaining sage. Mash chopped sage, garlic, ½ teaspoon salt and ½ teaspoon pepper in small bowl to form paste. Stir in 2 tablepoons oil.

2 Score fatty side of pork with sharp knife, making cuts about ¼ inch deep. Rub herb paste into cuts and onto all sides of pork. Place pork on large plate; cover and refrigerate 1 to 2 hours.

3 Preheat oven to 400°F. Cut rutabaga into halves or quarters; peel and cut into 1½-inch pieces. Place rutabaga and carrots in large bowl. Drizzle with remaining 3 tablespoons oil and sprinkle with remaining 1 teaspoon salt and ½ teaspoon pepper; toss to coat.

4 Arrange vegetables in single layer in large roasting pan. Place pork on top of vegetables, scraping any remaining herb paste from plate into roasting pan. Tuck 3 sprigs of remaining sage into vegetables.

5 Roast 15 minutes. *Reduce oven temperature to 325°F.* Roast 45 minutes to 1 hour and 15 minutes or until 145°F and pork is barely pink in center, stirring vegetables once or twice during cooking time. Let pork stand 5 minutes before slicing.

Makes 4 to 6 servings

TIP: Rutabagas can be difficult to cut—they are a tough vegetable and slippery on the outside because they are waxed. Cutting them into large pieces (halves or quarters) before peeling and chopping makes them easier to manage.

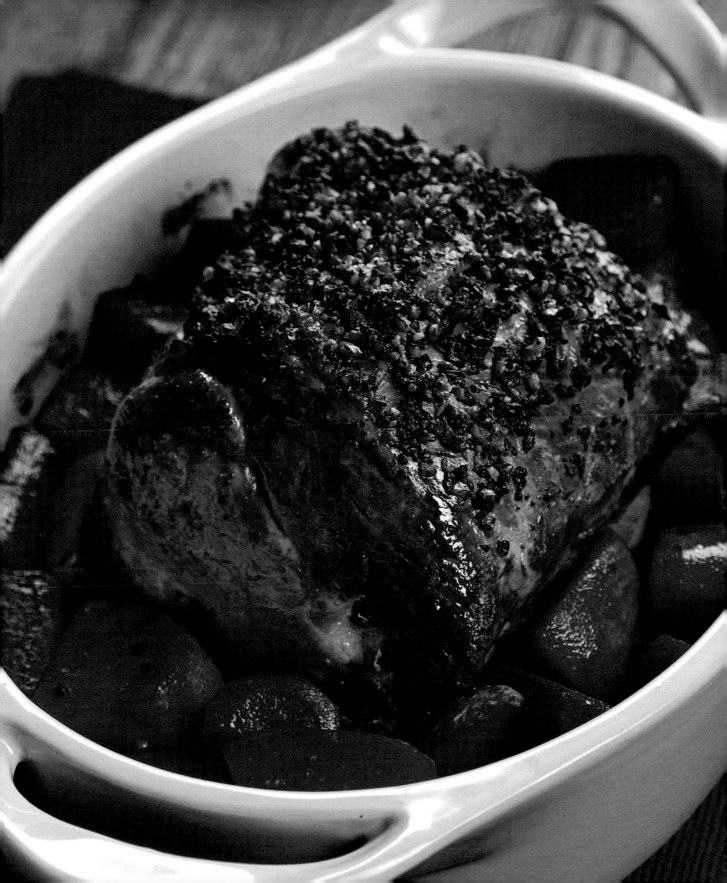

PORK TENDERLOIN WITH AVOCADO-TOMATILLO SALSA

1½ teaspoons chili powder

½ teaspoon ground cumin

1 pound pork tenderloin

1 tablespoon olive oil

2 medium tomatillos, husked and diced*

½ ripe medium avocado, diced

2 tablespoons finely chopped red onion

1 to 2 tablespoons chopped fresh cilantro

1 tablespoon lime juice

1 jalapeño pepper,** seeded and finely chopped

1 clove garlic, minced

⅛ teaspoon salt

4 lime wedges (optional)

Remove the husk by pulling from the bottom to where it attaches at the stem. Wash before using.

**Jalapeño peppers can sting and irritate the skin, so wear rubber gloves when handling and do not touch your eyes.*

1 Preheat oven to 425°F. Line rimmed baking sheet with foil.

2 Combine chili powder and cumin in small bowl. Sprinkle mixture over pork, pressing to adhere.

3 Heat oil in large skillet over medium-high heat until hot. Add pork; cook 3 minutes per side or until well browned. Place on prepared baking sheet.

4 Roast 20 to 25 minutes or until barely pink in center. Remove to cutting board; let stand 5 minutes before slicing.

5 Combine tomatillos, avocado, onion, cilantro, lime juice, jalapeño, garlic and salt in medium bowl; toss gently to blend. Serve pork with salsa and and lime wedges, if desired.

Makes 4 servings

TIP: Choose firm tomatillos with dry husks that are not too ragged. Store in a paper bag in the refrigerator for up to one month.

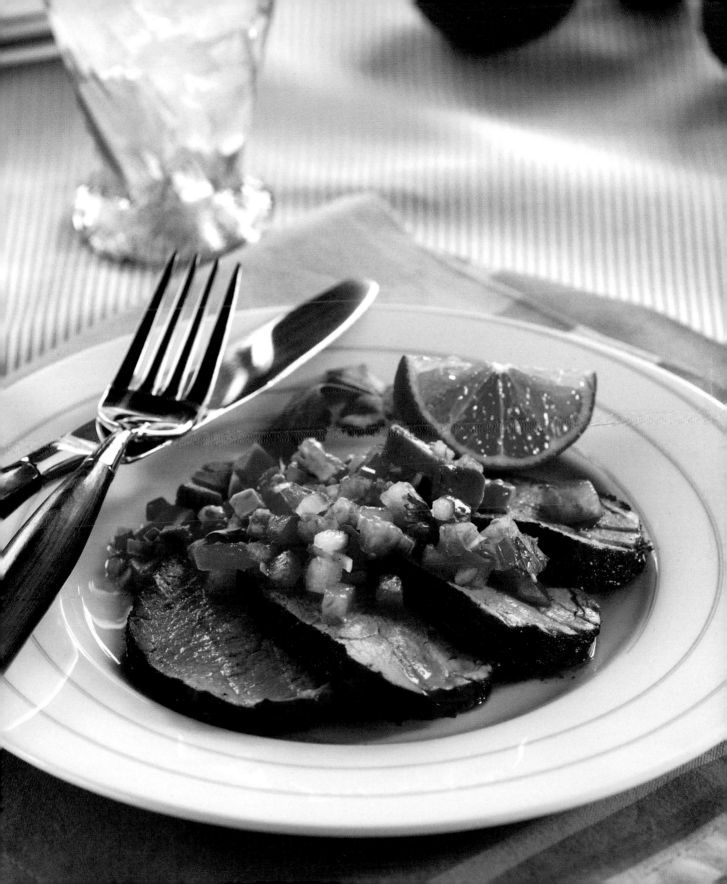

LAMB

ROSEMARY-GARLIC LAMB CHOPS

- 6 **cloves garlic**
- 1 **teaspoon salt**
- 2 **tablespoons finely chopped fresh rosemary leaves**
- 2 **tablespoons olive oil**
- ½ **teaspoon black pepper**
- 12 **small lamb rib chops, bone-in and frenched***

The term frenched means that the fat and meat have been cut away from the end of the bone protruding from the chop. Ask the butcher to do this for you if pre-cut frenched chops are not available. You can also purchase a frenched rack of lamb and cut it into individual chops.

1 Chop garlic with salt until finely minced. Place in small bowl. Add rosemary, oil and pepper; mix well.

2 Rub mixture on both sides of lamb chops; wrap in single layer in foil and refrigerate 30 minutes to 3 hours.

3 Oil grid. Prepare grill for direct cooking or preheat broiler. Grill lamb over medium-high heat 2 to 5 minutes per side or until medium-rare (145°F). Lamb should feel slightly firm when pressed. (To check doneness, cut small slit in meat near bone; lamb should be rosy pink.)

Makes 4 servings

VARIATION: Add 2 teaspoons Dijon mustard to the marinade.

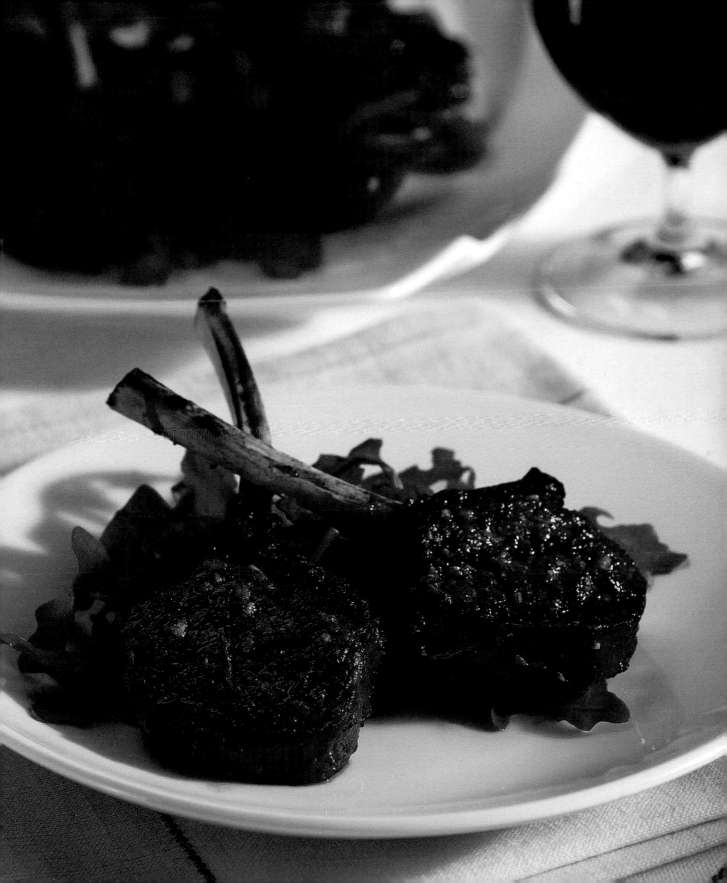

BRAISED LAMB SHANKS WITH ORANGE AND ROSEMARY

DRY RUB

1 teaspoon coarse salt
1 teaspoon paprika
1 teaspoon dried oregano
½ teaspoon black pepper
½ teaspoon ground cumin
⅛ teaspoon ground cloves

LAMB

4 lamb shanks (about 1 pound each)
2 tablespoons olive oil
1 large leek, cut into ½-inch pieces
2 carrots, cut into 1-inch pieces
2 stalks celery, cut into 1-inch pieces
1 medium bulb fennel, cut into ¼-inch slices
½ cup red wine
4 cups chicken broth
2 bay leaves
1 small bunch fresh thyme (about 6 stems)
1 sprig fresh rosemary
1 orange, cut into ¼-inch slices
½ teaspoon salt
¼ teaspoon black pepper

1 Combine coarse salt, oregano, paprika, pepper, cumin and cloves in small bowl; mix well. Rub mixture over lamb. Cover and marinate in refrigerator at least 1 hour or overnight.

2 Preheat oven to 350°F. Heat oil in Dutch oven over medium-high heat. Add leek; cook and stir until translucent. Add carrots, celery and fennel; cook and stir 5 minutes. Add wine; cook until reduced to about 1 tablespoon. Arrange lamb on top of vegetables. Add broth, bay leaves, thyme, rosemary and orange slices. If broth does not cover lamb, add just enough water to cover. Bring to a boil.

3 Reduce heat to low; cover and bake 1½ to 2 hours or until lamb is very tender and meat begins to fall off bone.

4 Remove lamb and vegetables from Dutch oven; keep warm. Remove and discard herbs. Skim fat from remaining liquid; simmer over medium heat 15 to 20 minutes or until liquid is reduced by half. Stir in salt and pepper. Serve sauce with lamb and vegetables.

Makes 4 servings

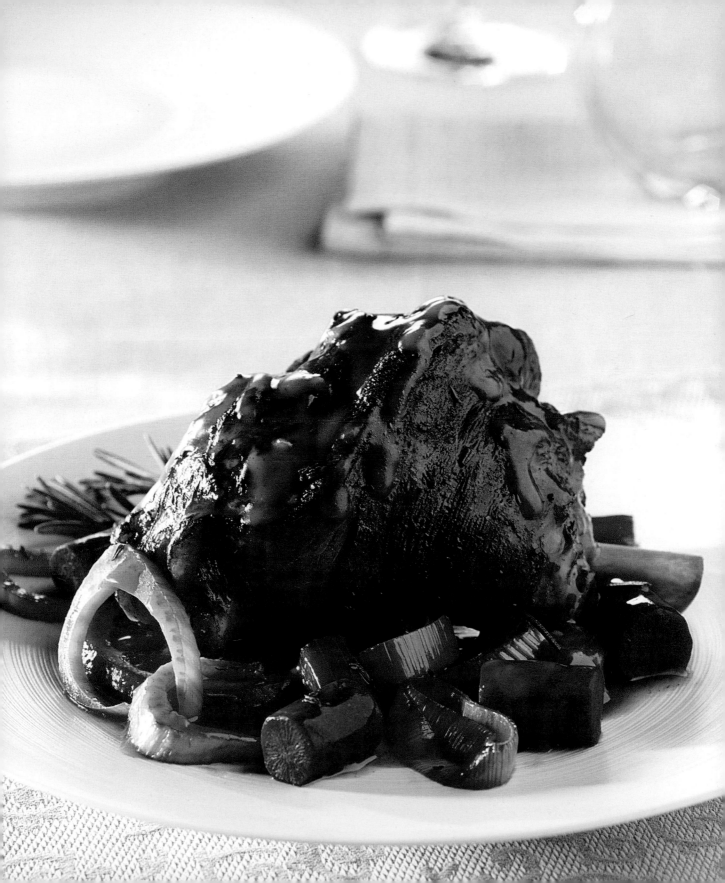

GREEK LEG OF LAMB

· · · · · · · · · · · · ·

2½ to 3 pounds boneless leg of lamb
¼ cup Dijon mustard
2 tablespoons minced fresh rosemary leaves
4 cloves garlic, minced
2 teaspoons salt
2 teaspoons black pepper
¼ cup olive oil

1 Untie and unroll lamb to lie flat; trim fat.

2 Combine mustard, rosemary, garlic, salt and pepper in small bowl; whisk in oil. Spread mixture evenly over lamb, coating both sides. Place lamb in large resealable food storage bag. Seal bag; refrigerate at least 2 hours or overnight, turning several times.

3 Prepare grill for direct cooking. Grill lamb over medium-high heat 35 to 40 minutes or to desired doneness. Transfer lamb to cutting board. Tent with foil; let stand 5 to 10 minutes before slicing. (Remove from grill at 140°F for medium. Temperature will rise 5°F while resting.)

Makes 6 to 8 servings

· · · · · · · · ·

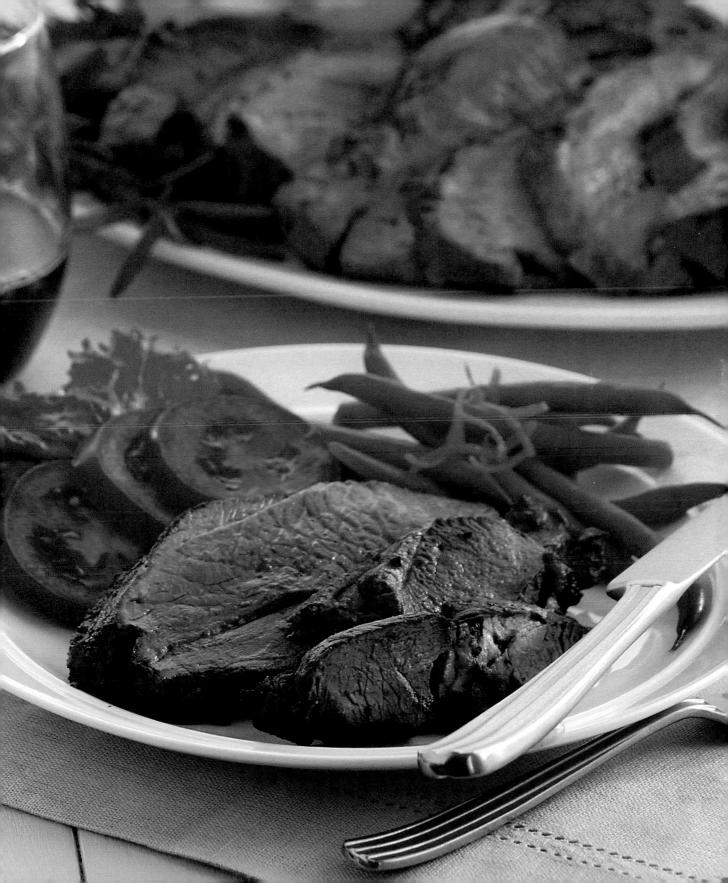

MOROCCAN-STYLE LAMB CHOPS

- 1 **tablespoon olive oil**
- 1 **teaspoon ground cumin**
- 1 **teaspoon ground coriander**
- ¾ **teaspoon salt**
- ⅛ **teaspoon ground cinnamon**
- ⅛ **teaspoon ground red pepper**
- 4 **center-cut lamb loin chops, 1 inch thick (about 4 ounces each)**
- 2 **cloves garlic, minced**

1 Prepare grill for direct cooking or preheat broiler. Combine oil, cumin, coriander, salt, cinnamon and red pepper in small bowl; mix well. Rub or brush mixture over both sides of lamb. Sprinkle garlic over both sides of lamb.

2 Grill lamb, covered, 5 minutes per side for medium doneness.

Makes 4 servings

ITALIAN TOMATO-BRAISED LAMB

- 4 **bone-in lamb shoulder chops, about 1 inch thick (about 10 ounces each)**
  Salt and black pepper
- 2 **onions, cut into quarters and thinly sliced**
- 1 **can (28 ounces) whole plum tomatoes, undrained**
- 2 **tablespoons olive oil**
- 2 **tablespoons red wine vinegar**
- 3 **cloves garlic, minced**
- 1½ **teaspoons dried oregano**
- 3 **to 4 sprigs fresh rosemary**

1 Preheat oven to 400°F. Place lamb in 13×9-inch baking dish; season with salt and pepper. Top with onions.

2 Place tomatoes with juice in medium bowl; break up tomatoes. Stir in oil, vinegar, garlic and oregano. Pour mixture over lamb and onions. Tuck rosemary sprigs into tomato mixture.

3 Cover and bake 45 minutes. Turn lamb and bake, uncovered, 1 hour and 15 minutes or until tender. Remove and discard rosemary sprigs.

Makes 4 servings

Moroccan-Style Lamb Chops

ROASTED DIJON LAMB WITH HERBS AND COUNTRY VEGETABLES

. . . .

4½ pounds boneless leg of lamb, trimmed
20 cloves garlic, peeled (about 2 medium heads)
¼ cup Dijon mustard
2 tablespoons water
2 tablespoons fresh rosemary leaves
1 tablespoon fresh thyme leaves
1¼ teaspoons salt, divided
1 teaspoon black pepper
1 pound parsnips, cut diagonally into ½-inch pieces
1 pound carrots, cut diagonally into ½-inch pieces
2 large onions, cut into ½-inch wedges
3 tablespoons extra virgin olive oil, divided

1 Place lamb in large resealable food storage bag. Combine garlic, mustard, water, rosemary, thyme, ¾ teaspoon salt and pepper in food processor; process until smooth. Spoon mixture over top and sides of lamb. Seal bag; refrigerate at least 8 hours.

2 Preheat oven to 500°F. Line broiler pan with foil; top with broiler rack. Combine parsnips, carrots, onions and 2 tablespoons oil in large bowl; toss to coat. Spread evenly on broiler rack; top with lamb.

3 Roast 15 minutes. *Reduce oven temperature to 325°F.* Roast 1 hour and 20 minutes until 145°F for medium or until desired doneness.

4 Transfer lamb to cutting board; let stand 10 minutes before slicing. Continue roasting vegetables 10 minutes.

5 Transfer vegetables to large bowl. Add remaining 1 tablespoon oil and ½ teaspoon salt; toss to coat. Thinly slice lamb; serve with vegetables.

Makes 8 to 10 servings

. . . .

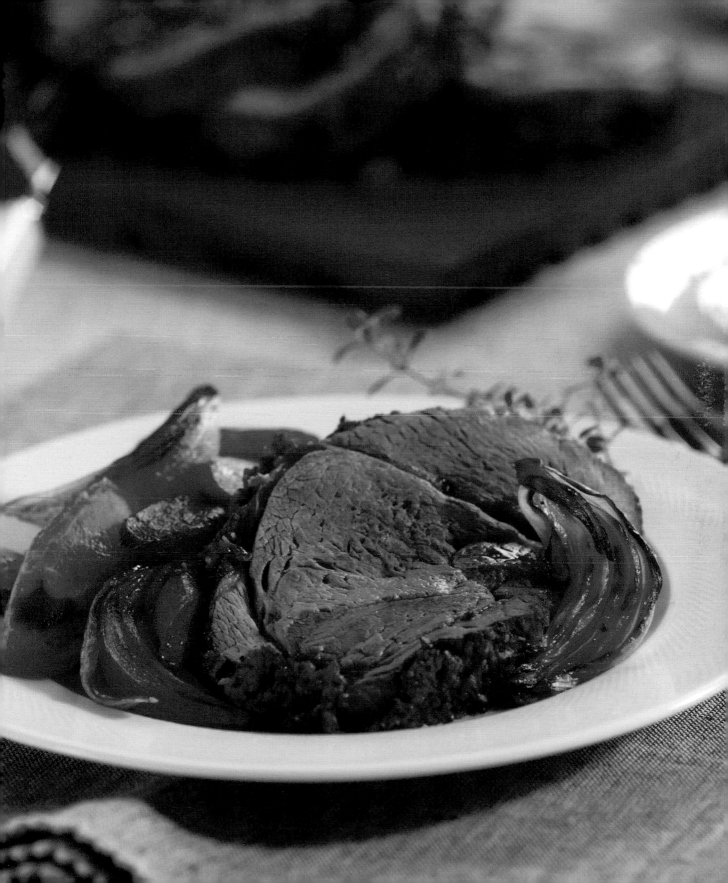

HERBED LAMB CHOPS

⅓ cup olive oil
⅓ cup red wine vinegar
2 tablespoons coconut aminos*
1 tablespoon lemon juice
3 cloves garlic, minced
1 teaspoon salt
1 teaspoon chopped fresh oregano *or* ¼ teaspoon dried oregano
1 teaspoon dried rosemary
1 teaspoon ground mustard
½ teaspoon white pepper
8 lamb loin chops, 1 inch thick (about 4 ounces each)

*Coconut aminos is a dark, salty soy-free sauce containing 17 amino acids. It is made from the sap of the coconut tree which is dried and blended with sea salt. It does not have a pronounced coconut flavor and is often used as a substitute for soy sauce in paleo recipes. Coconut aminos can be found in health food and vitamin stores, some grocery stores or online.

1 Combine all ingredients except lamb in large resealable food storage bag. Reserve ½ cup marinade in small bowl. Add lamb to remaining marinade. Seal bag; turn to coat. Marinate in refrigerator at least 1 hour.

2 Prepare grill for direct cooking.

3 Remove lamb from marinade; discard marinade. Grill lamb over medium-high heat 8 minutes or to desired doneness, turning once and basting often with reserved ½ cup marinade. Do not baste during last 5 minutes of cooking. Discard any remaining marinade.

Makes 4 to 6 servings

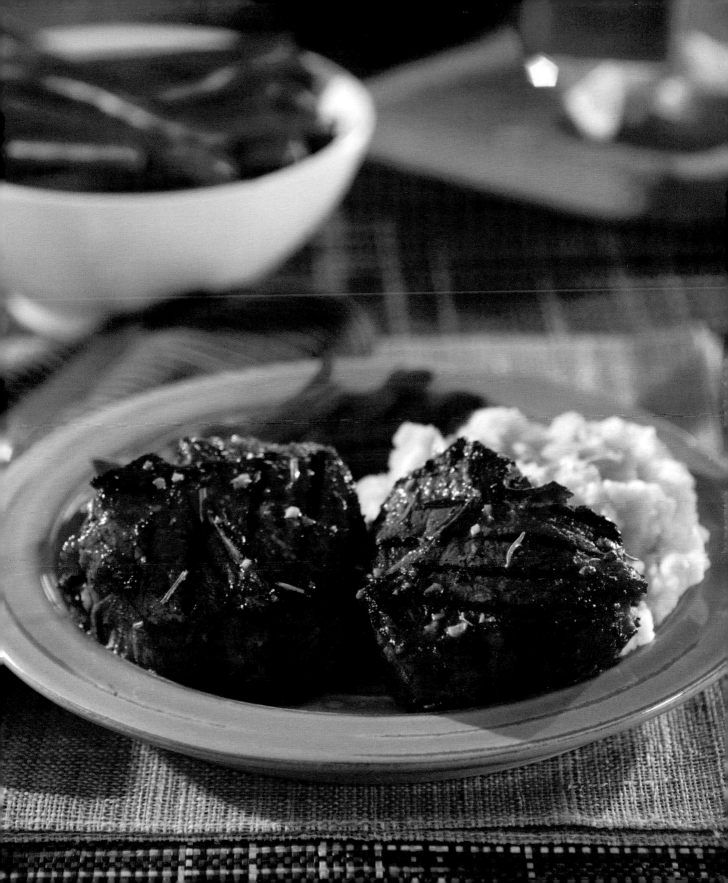

DELUXE MEDITERRANEAN LAMB BURGERS

1½ **pounds ground lamb**
1 **tablespoon minced garlic**
2 **teaspoons Greek seasoning**
1 **teaspoon paprika**
½ **teaspoon salt, divided**
½ **teaspoon black pepper**
4 **thin slices red onion, separated into rings**
1 **tablespoon olive oil**
1 **teaspoon chopped fresh mint or parsley**
1 **teaspoon red wine vinegar**
   Spinach leaves
4 **to 8 tomato slices**

1 Oil grid. Prepare grill for direct cooking.

2 Combine lamb, garlic, Greek seasoning, paprika, ¼ teaspoon salt and pepper in large bowl; mix lightly but thoroughly. Shape into four patties about ¾ inch thick. Cover and refrigerate.

3 Combine onion, oil, mint, vinegar and remaining ¼ teaspoon salt in small bowl; toss to coat.

4 Grill patties, covered, over medium heat 8 to 10 minutes (or uncovered, 13 to 15 minutes) until cooked through (160°F) or until desired doneness, turning occasionally.

5 Serve burgers over spinach; top with tomatoes and onion mixture.

Makes 4 servings

SERBIAN LAMB SAUSAGE KABOBS

1 **pound lean ground lamb**
1 **pound ground beef**
1 **small onion, finely chopped**
1 **egg, lightly beaten**
1 **tablespoon hot Hungarian paprika**
2 **cloves garlic, minced**
   Salt and black pepper
3 **to 4 red, green or yellow bell peppers, cut into squares**

1 Combine lamb, beef, onion, egg, paprika and garlic in large bowl; mix well. Season with salt and black pepper.

2 Place meat mixture on cutting board; pat evenly into 8×6-inch rectangle. Cut meat into 48 (1-inch) squares with sharp knife; shape each square into small oblong sausage.

3 Place sausages on waxed paper-lined jelly-roll pan; freeze 30 to 45 minutes or until firm. (Do not freeze completely.) Meanwhile, prepare grill for direct cooking.

4 Alternately thread sausages and bell pepper pieces onto metal skewers.

5 Grill kabobs over medium-high heat 5 to 7 minutes. Turn and grill 5 to 7 minutes or until meat is cooked through.

Makes 8 servings

NOTE: The seasonings can be adjusted, but the key to authenticity is the equal parts of beef and lamb and the garlic and paprika. Try sweet paprika for a milder flavor.

FISH

GRILLED SWORDFISH SICILIAN STYLE

- 3 tablespoons extra virgin olive oil
- 1 clove garlic, minced
- 2 tablespoons lemon juice
- ¾ teaspoon salt
- ⅛ teaspoon black pepper
- 3 tablespoons capers, drained
- 1 tablespoon chopped fresh oregano or basil
- 4 swordfish steaks, ¾ inch thick (about 6 ounces each)

1 Oil grid. Prepare grill for direct cooking.

2 Heat oil in small saucepan over low heat. Add garlic; cook 1 minute. Remove from heat; cool slightly. Whisk in lemon juice, salt and pepper until salt is dissolved. Stir in capers and oregano.

3 Grill swordfish over medium heat 7 to 8 minutes or until center is opaque, turning once. Serve with sauce.

Makes 4 to 6 servings

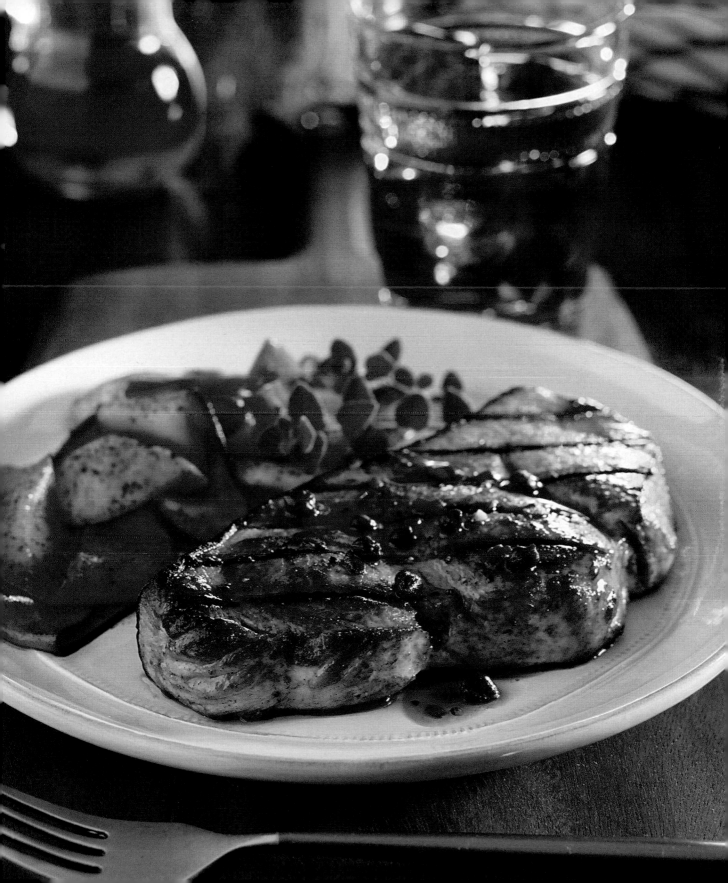

GREEK-STYLE SALMON

· · · · · · · · · · · · · · · · ·

  1½ **tablespoons olive oil**
  1¾ **cups diced tomatoes, drained**
    6 **pitted black olives, coarsely chopped**
    4 **pitted green olives, coarsely chopped**
    3 **tablespoons lemon juice**
    2 **tablespoons chopped fresh Italian parsley**
    1 **tablespoon capers, rinsed and drained**
    2 **cloves garlic, thinly sliced**
   ¼ **teaspoon black pepper**
    4 **salmon fillets (4 to 6 ounces each)**

1 Heat oil in large skillet over medium heat. Add tomatoes, olives, lemon juice, parsley, capers, garlic and pepper; bring to a simmer, stirring frequently. Simmer 5 minutes or until reduced by about one third, stirring occasionally.

2 Rinse salmon and pat dry with paper towels. Push sauce to one side of skillet. Add fish to skillet; spoon sauce over fish. Cover and cook 10 to 15 minutes or until fish begins to flake when tested with fork.

Makes 4 servings

· · · · · · · ·

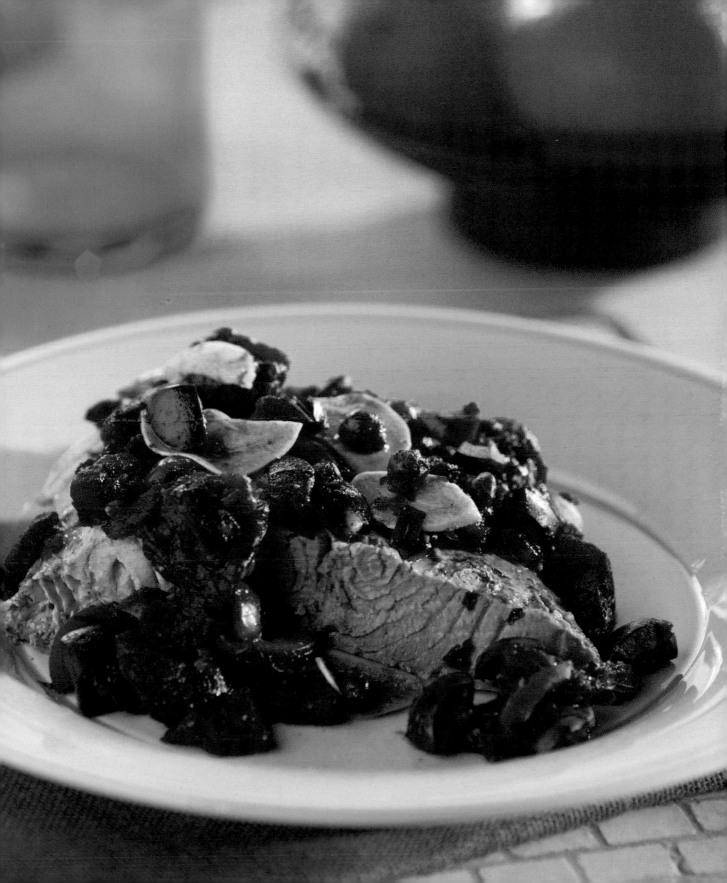

BROILED COD WITH SALSA SALAD

- 2 tablespoons olive oil, divided, plus additional for pan
- 1 green bell pepper, diced
- 2 medium tomatoes, chopped
- ½ cup chopped red onion
- 1 serrano chile pepper,* minced
- 1 tablespoon chopped fresh cilantro
- 1 teaspoon white wine vinegar
- ½ teaspoon salt, divided
- ½ teaspoon black pepper, divided
- ⅛ teaspoon dried oregano
- 4 cod fillets, about ¾ inch thick (3 to 4 ounces each)
- 4 lemon wedges

Serrano chile peppers can sting and irritate the skin, so wear rubber gloves when handling peppers and do not touch your eyes.

1 Preheat broiler. Brush shallow baking pan with oil.

2 Combine bell pepper, tomatoes, onion, serrano pepper, cilantro, 1 tablespoon oil, vinegar, ¼ teaspoon salt and ¼ teaspoon black pepper in large bowl; toss to coat.

3 Combine remaining 1 tablespoon oil, ¼ teaspoon salt, ¼ teaspoon black pepper and oregano in small bowl; mix well. Place cod in prepared pan; brush with spice mixture.

4 Broil 4 inches from heat source 6 to 8 minutes or until fish begins to flake when tested with fork. Serve with salad; garnish with lemon wedges.

Makes 4 servings

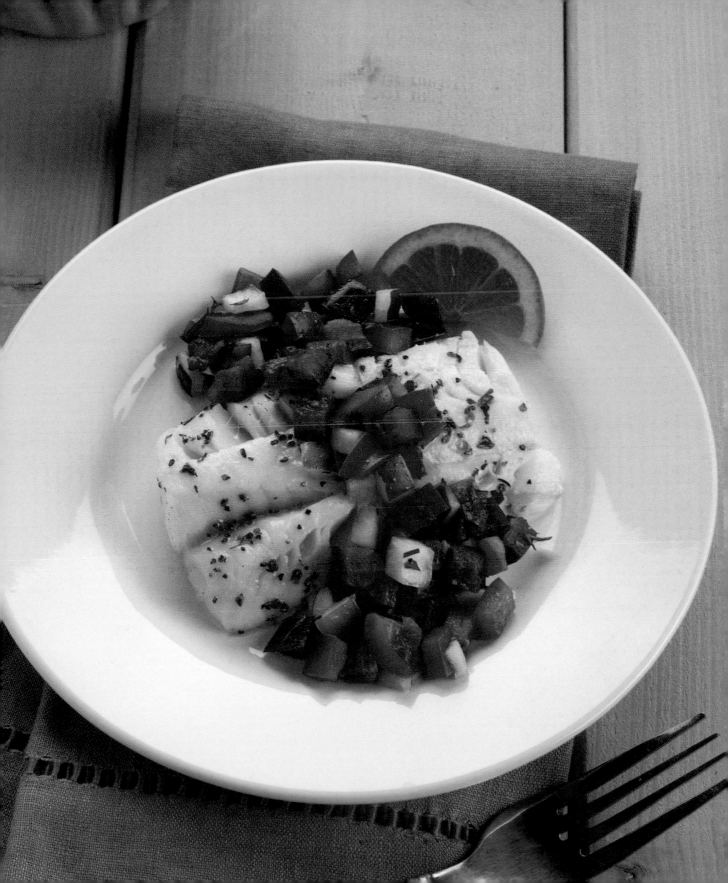

SALMON SALAD WITH BASIL VINAIGRETTE

Basil Vinaigrette (recipe follows)
1½ teaspoons salt, divided
1 pound asparagus, trimmed
4 salmon fillets (4 to 6 ounces each)
1 tablespoon olive oil
¼ teaspoon black pepper
4 lemon wedges

1 Prepare Basil Vinaigrette. Preheat oven to 400°F or prepare grill for direct cooking.

2 Combine 3 inches of water and 1 teaspoon salt in large saucepan; bring to boil over high heat. Add asparagus; simmer 6 to 8 minutes or until crisp-tender. Drain and set aside.

3 Brush salmon with oil; sprinkle with remaining ½ teaspoon salt and pepper. Place fish in shallow baking pan; bake 11 to 13 minutes or until center is opaque. (Or grill on well-oiled grid over medium-high heat 4 or 5 minutes per side or until center is opaque.)

4 Remove skin from fish; break into bite-size pieces. Arrange fish over asparagus; drizzle with Basil Vinaigrette. Serve with lemon wedges.

Makes 4 servings

BASIL VINAIGRETTE

3 tablespoons extra virgin olive oil
1 tablespoon white wine vinegar
1 tablespoon minced fresh basil
1 clove garlic, minced
1 teaspoon minced fresh chives
¼ teaspoon black pepper
⅛ teaspoon salt

Combine all ingredients in small bowl; mix well.

Makes about ¼ cup

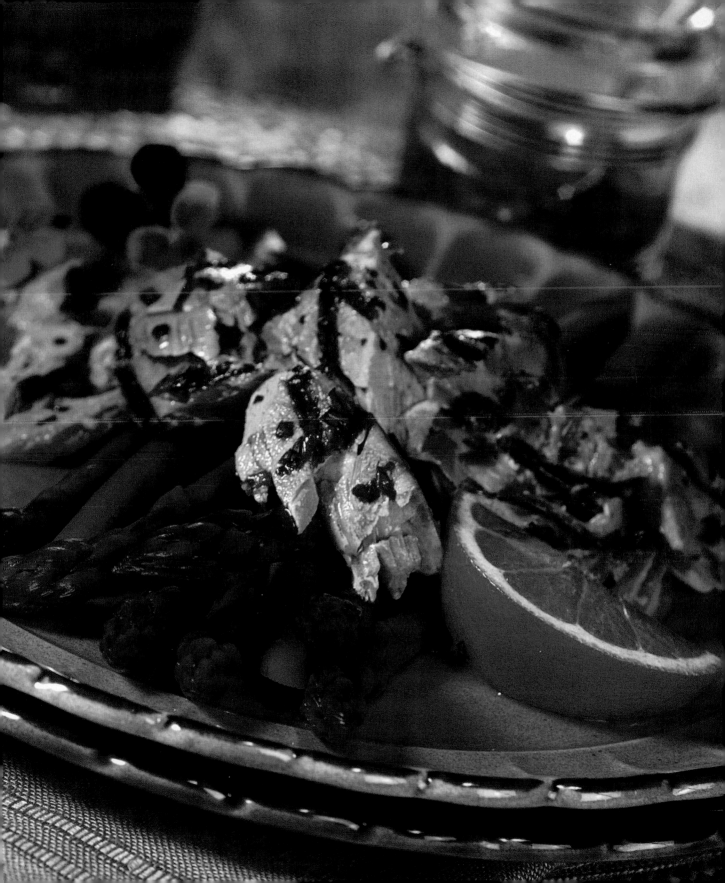

MUSTARD-GRILLED RED SNAPPER

  ½ cup Dijon mustard
  1 tablespoon red wine vinegar
  1 teaspoon ground red pepper
  ¼ teaspoon salt
  4 red snapper fillets (about 6 ounces each)

1 Oil grid. Prepare grill for direct cooking.

2 Combine mustard, vinegar, red pepper and salt in small bowl; mix well. Coat snapper thoroughly with mustard mixture.

3 Grill fish, covered, over medium-high heat 4 minutes per side or until fish begins to flake when tested with fork.

Makes 4 servings

ADRIATIC-STYLE HALIBUT

  1 large tomato, seeded and diced (about 1¼ cups)
  ⅓ cup coarsely chopped pitted kalamata olives
  1 clove garlic, minced
  4 skinless halibut or red snapper fillets (about 6 ounces each)
  ¾ teaspoon coarse salt
  ¼ teaspoon black pepper
  1 tablespoon olive oil
  ¼ cup white wine
  2 tablespoons chopped fresh basil or Italian parsley

1 Preheat oven to 200°F. Combine tomato, olives and garlic in small bowl; mix well. Sprinkle halibut with salt and pepper.

2 Heat oil in large nonstick skillet over medium heat. Add fish; cook 8 to 10 minutes or just until center is opaque, turning once. Transfer to serving platter; keep warm in oven.

3 Add wine to skillet; cook over high heat until reduced to 2 tablespoons. Add tomato mixture; cook and stir 1 to 2 minutes or until heated through. Season with additional salt and pepper. Spoon tomato mixture over fish; sprinkle with basil.

Makes 4 servings

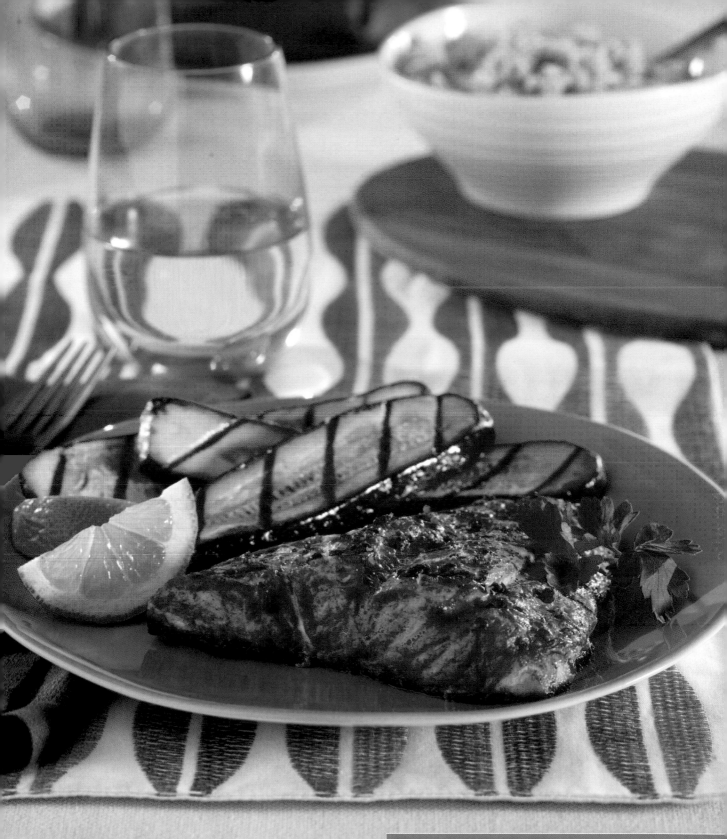

Mustard-Grilled Red Snapper

HALIBUT WITH ROASTED PEPPER SAUCE

Roasted Pepper Sauce (recipe follows)
1   teaspoon olive oil
1   medium onion, thinly sliced
1   clove garlic, minced
1   halibut fillet (1½ pounds), skinned

1 Preheat oven to 425°F. Prepare Roasted Pepper Sauce.

2 Brush shallow baking dish with oil. Scatter onion and garlic over bottom of dish; top with halibut and sauce.

3 Bake 20 minutes or until fish flakes begins to flake when tested with fork.

Makes 4 servings

ROASTED PEPPER SAUCE

1   can (7 ounces) chopped green chiles, drained
1   jar (7 ounces) roasted red peppers, drained
⅔   cup chicken broth
¼   teaspoon salt

Combine chiles, roasted peppers, broth and salt in food processor or blender; process until smooth.

Makes about ¾ cup

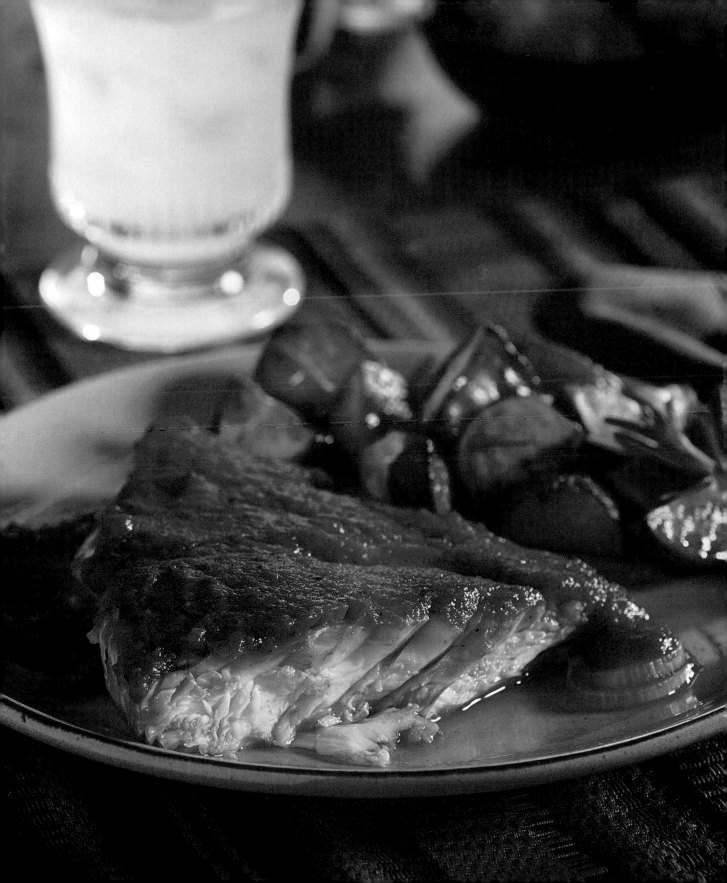

TUNA STEAKS WITH PINEAPPLE AND TOMATO SALSA

- 1 medium tomato, chopped
- 1 cup chopped pineapple
- 2 tablespoons chopped fresh cilantro
- 1 jalapeño pepper,* seeded and minced
- 1 tablespoon minced red onion
- 2 teaspoons lime juice
- ½ teaspoon grated lime peel
- 4 tuna steaks (about 4 ounces each)
- ½ teaspoon salt
- ⅛ teaspoon black pepper
- 1 tablespoon olive oil

Jalapeño peppers can sting and irritate the skin, so wear rubber gloves when handling peppers and do not touch your eyes.

1 Combine tomato, pineapple, cilantro, jalapeño, onion, lime juice and lime peel in medium bowl; mix well.

2 Sprinkle tuna with salt and pepper. Heat oil in large nonstick skillet over medium-high heat. Add fish; cook 2 to 3 minutes per side for medium-rare or until desired doneness. Serve with salsa.

Makes 4 servings

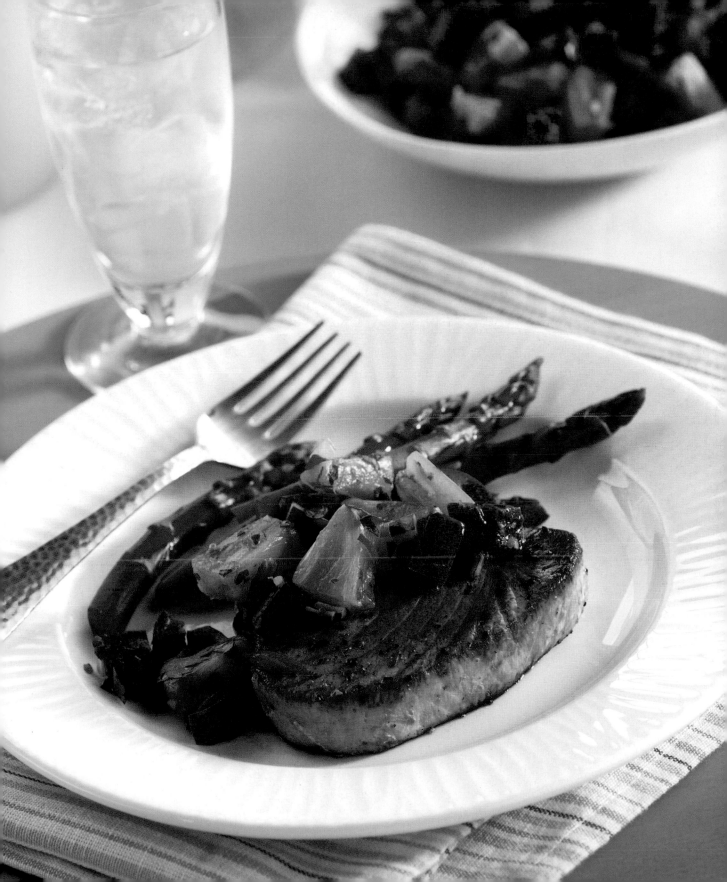

DILLED SALMON IN PARCHMENT

2 skinless salmon fillets (4 to 6 ounces each)
2 tablespoons butter, melted
1 tablespoon lemon juice
1 tablespoon chopped fresh dill
1 tablespoon chopped shallots
   Salt and black pepper

1 Preheat oven to 400°F. Cut 2 pieces of parchment paper into 12-inch squares; fold squares in half diagonally and cut into half heart shapes. Open parchment; place fish fillet on one side of each heart.

2 Combine butter and lemon juice in small cup; drizzle over fish. Sprinkle with dill, shallots and salt and pepper to taste. Fold parchment hearts in half. Beginning at top of heart, fold edges together, 2 inches at a time. At tip of heart, fold parchment over to seal.

3 Bake fish about 10 minutes or until parchment pouch puffs up. To serve, cut an "X" through top layer of parchment and fold back points.

Makes 2 servings

BROILED HUNAN FISH FILLETS

3 tablespoons coconut aminos
1 tablespoon finely chopped green onion
2 teaspoons dark sesame oil
1 clove garlic, minced
1 teaspoon minced fresh ginger
¼ teaspoon red pepper flakes
4 red snapper, scrod or cod fillets (5 to 7 ounces each)

1 Preheat broiler. Oil rack of broiler pan. Combine coconut aminos, green onion, oil, garlic, ginger and red pepper flakes in small bowl; mix well.

2 Place snapper on prepared broiler rack; brush with green onion mixture.

3 Broil 4 to 5 inches from heat 10 minutes or until fish begins to flake when tested with fork.

Makes 4 servings

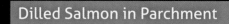
Dilled Salmon in Parchment

GRILLED RED SNAPPER WITH AVOCADO-PAPAYA SALSA

- 1 teaspoon ground coriander
- 1 teaspoon paprika
- ¾ teaspoon salt
- ⅛ to ¼ teaspoon ground red pepper
- ½ cup diced ripe avocado
- ½ cup diced ripe papaya
- 2 tablespoons chopped fresh cilantro
- 1 tablespoon lime juice
- 4 skinless red snapper or halibut fillets (5 to 7 ounces each)
- 1 tablespoon olive oil
- 4 lime wedges

1 Oil grid. Prepare grill for direct cooking. Combine coriander, paprika, salt and red pepper in small bowl; mix well.

2 Combine avocado, papaya, cilantro, lime juice and ¼ teaspoon spice mixture in medium bowl; mix well.

3 Brush oil over snapper; sprinkle with remaining spice mixture. Grill fish, covered, over medium-high heat 5 minutes per side or until fish begins to flake when tested with fork. Serve with salsa and lime wedges.

Makes 4 servings

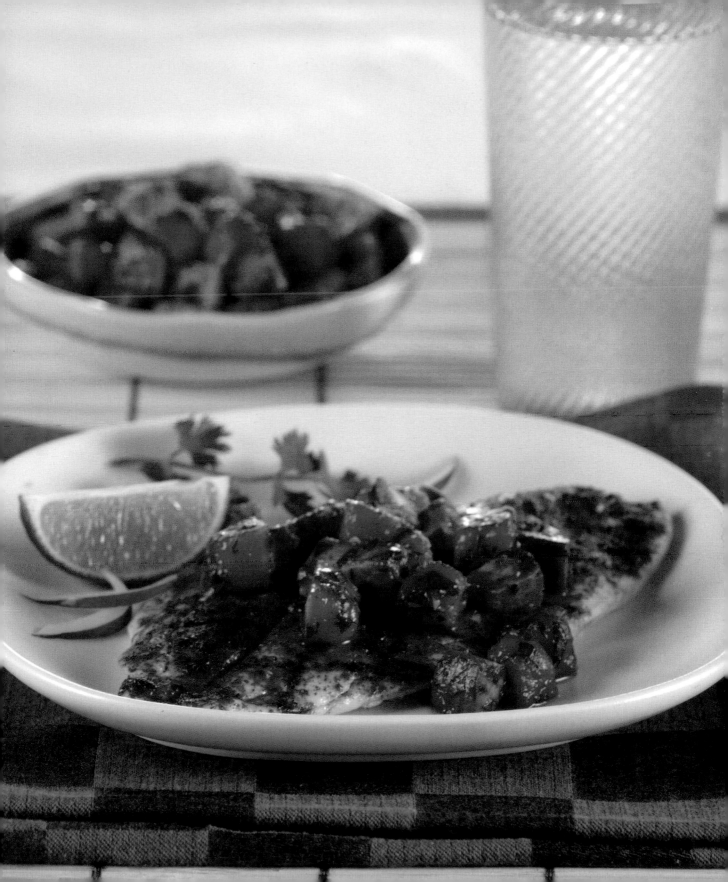

ROASTED DILL SCROD WITH ASPARAGUS

- 1 **bunch asparagus spears (about 12 ounces), trimmed**
- 1 **tablespoon olive oil**
- 4 **scrod or cod fillets (about 5 ounces each)**
- 1 **tablespoon lemon juice**
- 1 **teaspoon dried dill weed**
- ½ **teaspoon salt**
- ¼ **teaspoon black pepper**
  - **Paprika (optional)**

1 Preheat oven to 425°F. Place asparagus in 13×9-inch baking dish; drizzle with oil. Roll asparagus to coat lightly with oil; push to edges of dish, stacking asparagus into two layers.

2 Arrange scrod in center of dish; drizzle with lemon juice. Combine dill, salt and pepper in small bowl; sprinkle over fish and asparagus. Sprinkle with paprika, if desired.

3 Roast 15 to 17 minutes or until asparagus is crisp-tender and fish begins to flake when tested with fork.

Makes 4 servings

GROUPER SCAMPI

- 3 **tablespoons butter, softened**
- 1 **tablespoon white wine**
- 1 **teaspoon minced garlic**
- ½ **teaspoon grated lemon peel**
- ¼ **teaspoon salt**
- ⅛ **teaspoon black pepper**
- 4 **grouper, red snapper or orange roughy fillets (4 to 5 ounces each)**

1 Preheat oven to 450°F. Line shallow baking pan with foil.

2 Combine butter, wine, garlic, lemon peel, salt and pepper in small bowl; mix well. Place grouper in prepared pan; top with butter mixture.

3 Bake 10 to 12 minutes or until fish begins to flake when tested with fork.

Makes 4 servings

Roasted Dill Scrod with Asparagus

WARM BLACKENED TUNA SALAD

- 1 teaspoon olive oil, plus additional for pan
- 5 cups torn romaine lettuce
- 2 cups coarsely shredded red cabbage
- 2 medium yellow or green bell peppers, cut into strips
- 1½ cups sliced zucchini
- 1 teaspoon onion powder
- ½ teaspoon garlic powder
- ½ teaspoon dried thyme
- ½ teaspoon ground red pepper
- ½ teaspoon black pepper
- 12 ounces tuna steaks, 1 inch thick
- ⅓ cup water
- ¾ cup sliced onion
- 2 tablespoons balsamic vinegar
- 1½ teaspoons Dijon mustard
- 1 teaspoon olive oil
- ¼ teaspoon salt

1 Preheat broiler. Brush broiler pan with oil. Combine romaine, cabbage, bell peppers and zucchini in large bowl; set aside.

2 Combine onion powder, garlic powder, thyme, ground red pepper and black pepper in small bowl; mix well. Rub spice mixture onto both sides of tuna. Place fish on prepared broiler pan.

3 Broil 4 inches from heat about 5 minutes per side or until desired doneness. Cover and set aside.

4 Bring water to a boil in small saucepan over high heat. Stir in onion. Reduce heat to medium-low; cover and simmer about 5 minutes or until onion is tender. Add vinegar, mustard, 1 teaspoon oil and salt; cook and stir until heated through.

5 Divide salad among four plates; slice tuna and place on salads. Drizzle with dressing. Serve warm.

Makes 4 servings

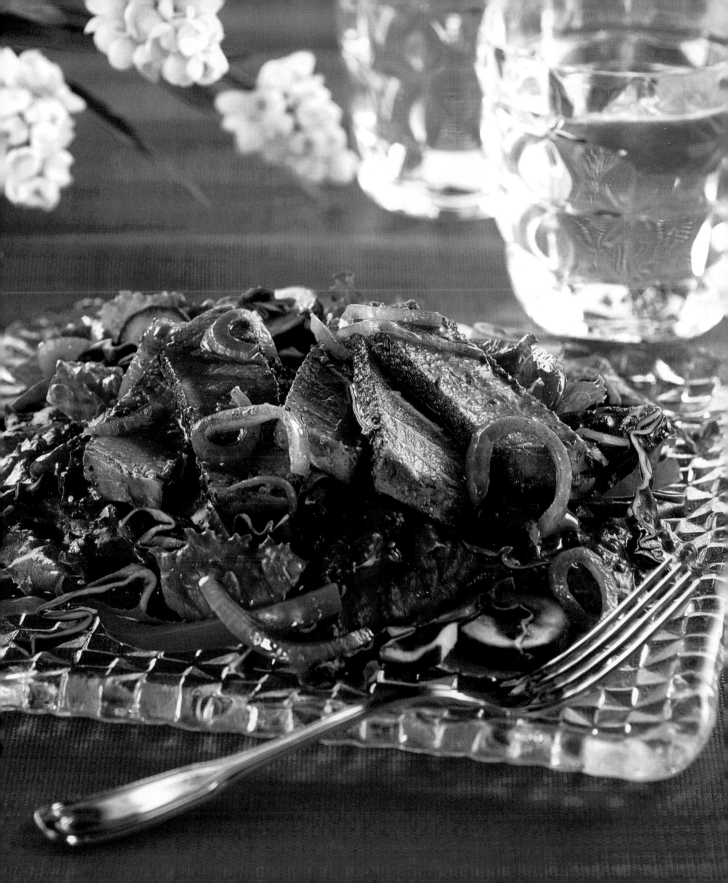

BAKED ORANGE ROUGHY WITH VEGETABLES

- 2 orange roughy fillets (about 4 ounces each)
- 1 tablespoon olive oil
- 1 medium carrot, cut into matchstick-size pieces
- 4 medium mushrooms, sliced
- ⅓ cup chopped onion
- ¼ cup chopped green or yellow bell pepper
- 1 clove garlic, minced
  Salt and black pepper
  Lemon wedges

1 Preheat oven to 350°F. Place orange roughy in shallow baking dish. Bake 15 minutes or until fish begins to flake when tested with fork.

2 Meanwhile, heat oil in medium skillet over medium-high heat. Add carrot; cook and stir 3 minutes. Add mushrooms, onion, bell pepper and garlic; cook and stir 5 minutes or until vegetables are crisp-tender.

3 Place fish on serving plates; top with vegetable mixture. Season with salt and black pepper. Serve with lemon wedges.

Makes 2 servings

VARIATION: To microwave fish, place fish in shallow microwavable dish. Microwave, covered, on HIGH 2 minutes or until fish begins to flake when tested with fork. To broil fish, place fish on rack of broiler pan. Broil 4 to 6 inches from heat 4 minutes per side or until fish begins to flake when tested with fork.

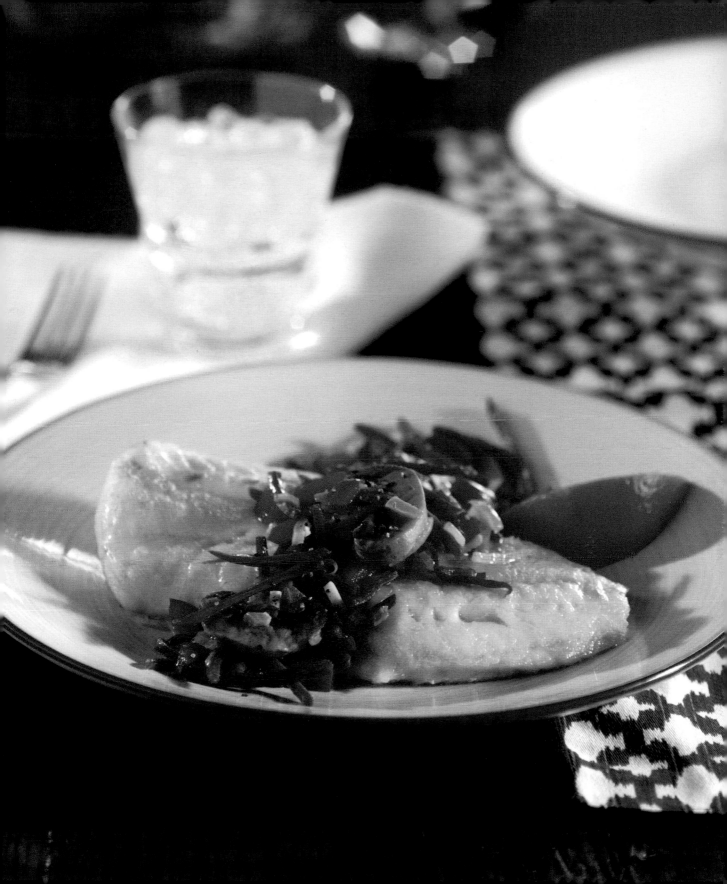

EASY HALIBUT STEAKS WITH TOMATO AND BROCCOLI SAUCE

- 2 tablespoons olive oil
- 2 cups chopped fresh broccoli
- 2½ cups diced fresh tomatoes
- 2 tablespoons lemon juice
- 1 tablespoon chopped garlic
- 1 tablespoon chopped fresh tarragon *or* 1 teaspoon dried tarragon
- ½ teaspoon salt
- ½ teaspoon black pepper
- 4 halibut steaks (about 4 ounces each)
- Lemon wedges (optional)

1 Heat oil in large skillet over medium heat. Add broccoli; cook and stir 5 minutes. Add tomatoes, lemon juice, garlic, tarragon, salt and pepper; cook and stir 5 minutes.

2 Add halibut to skillet; cover and cook 10 minutes or until fish is begins to flake when tested with fork.

3 Divide vegetables evenly among four plates; top with fish. Serve with lemon wedges, if desired.

Makes 4 servings

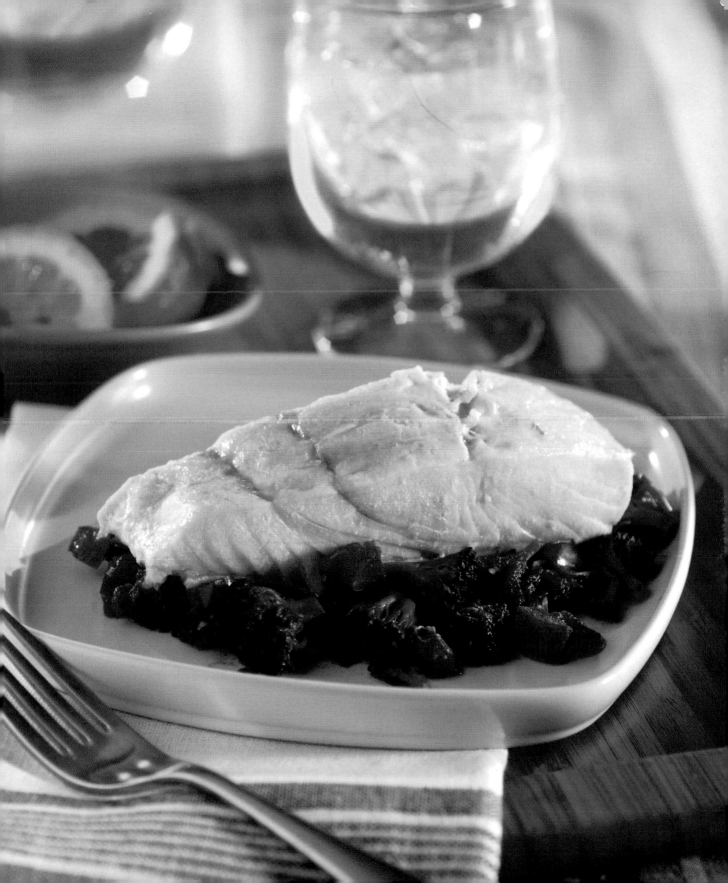

SPICED SALMON WITH PINEAPPLE-GINGER SALSA

· · · · · · · · · · · · · · · · · · · ·

- 1 tablespoon olive oil, plus additional for pan
- 1 teaspoon ground cumin
- ½ teaspoon salt
- ½ teaspoon ground allspice
- ¼ teaspoon black pepper
- 4 salmon steaks (4 to 6 ounces each), rinsed and patted dry
- ¾ cup finely chopped fresh pineapple
- ¼ cup finely chopped poblano pepper
- 2 tablespoons chopped cilantro
- 1 tablespoon lime juice
- 1 teaspoon grated fresh ginger
- ½ teaspoon grated orange peel

1 Preheat oven to 350°F. Brush baking sheet with oil.

2 Combine cumin, salt, allspice and black pepper in small bowl; mix well. Brush salmon with 1 tablespoon oil; sprinkle both sides of fish with spice mixture. Place on prepared baking sheet.

3 Bake fish 14 to 16 minutes or until center is opaque.

4 Meanwhile, combine pineapple, poblano, cilantro, lime juice, ginger and orange peel in medium bowl; mix well. Serve salsa with fish.

Makes 4 servings

· · · · · · · · ·

TIP: Store fresh unpeeled ginger tightly wrapped in the refrigerator for up to 2 weeks.

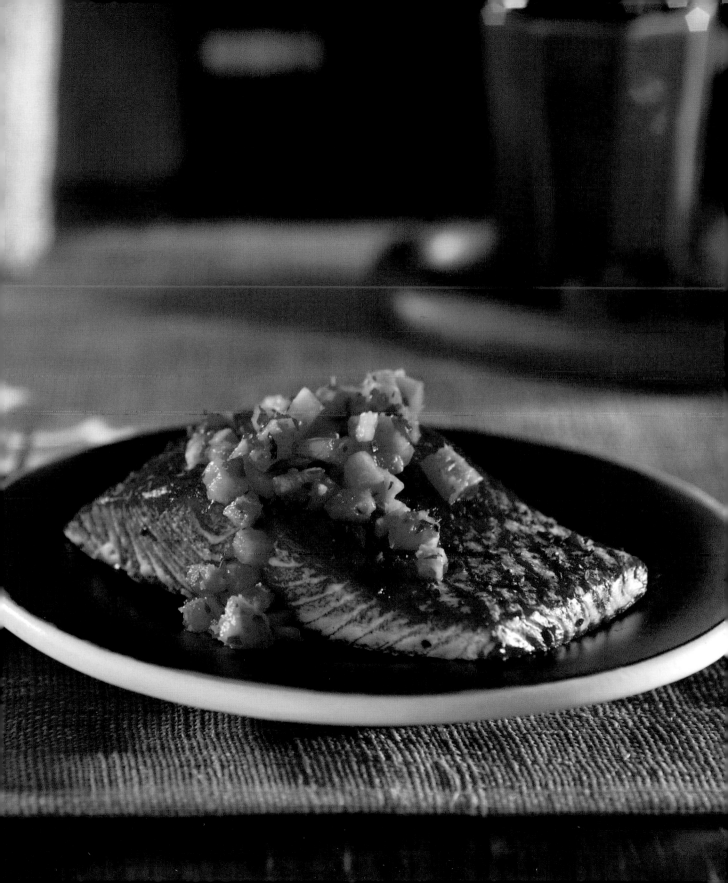

SHELLFISH

SHRIMP AND VEGGIE SKILLET TOSS

- ¼ cup coconut aminos
- 2 tablespoons lime juice
- 1 tablespoon dark sesame oil
- 1 teaspoon grated fresh ginger
- ⅛ teaspoon red pepper flakes
- 1 tablespoon olive oil, divided
- 8 ounces medium raw shrimp, peeled and deveined (with tails on)
- 2 medium zucchini, cut in half lengthwise and sliced
- 6 green onions, trimmed and halved lengthwise
- 12 grape tomatoes

1 Combine coconut aminos, lime juice, sesame oil, ginger and red pepper flakes in small bowl; mix well.

2 Heat half of olive oil in large nonstick skillet over medium-high heat. Add shrimp; cook and stir 3 minutes or until shrimp are opaque. Remove from skillet.

3 Heat remaining olive oil in same skillet. Add zucchini; cook and stir 4 to 6 minutes or just until crisp-tender. Add green onions and tomatoes; cook and stir 2 minutes. Add shrimp; cook 1 minute or until heated through. Remove to large bowl.

4 Add sauce to skillet; bring to a boil. Remove from heat. Stir in shrimp and vegetables; toss gently to coat.

Makes 4 servings

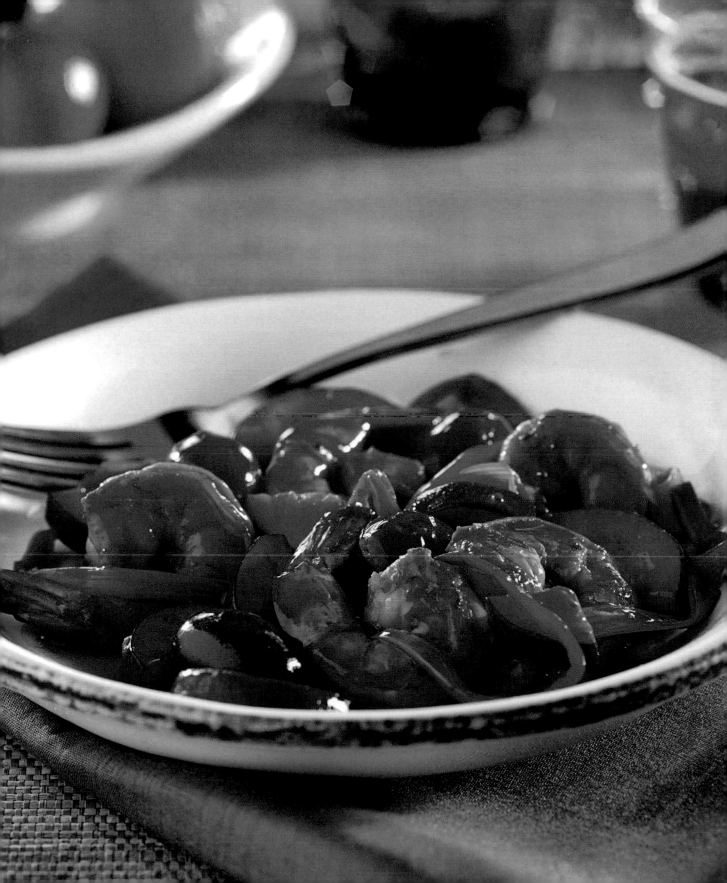

BASIL-LIME SCALLOPS

. . . .

  2 **tablespoons chopped fresh basil**
     Juice of 1 lime
  1 **tablespoon plus 1 teaspoon olive oil, divided**
  1 **teaspoon coconut aminos**
  1 **clove garlic, minced**
  ⅛ **teaspoon red pepper flakes**
  8 **jumbo sea scallops (about 1 pound)**
     Mixed baby greens and lime wedges (optional)

1 Whisk basil, lime juice, 1 teaspoon oil, coconut amimos, garlic and red pepper flakes in shallow bowl until well blended. Add scallops; turn to coat. Cover and marinate in refrigerator 30 minutes.

2 Heat remaining 1 tablespoon oil in large nonstick skillet over medium-high heat. Add scallops; cook 3 minutes per side or until scallops are opaque. Serve with mixed greens and lime wedges, if desired.

Makes 4 servings

. . . .

LEMON AND GARLIC SHRIMP

. . . .

  ¼ **cup olive oil**
  1 **pound large raw shrimp, peeled and deveined**
  3 **cloves garlic, crushed**
  2 **tablespoons lemon juice**
  ½ **teaspoon salt**
  ½ **teaspoon paprika**
     Black pepper
  2 **tablespoons finely chopped fresh parsley**

1 Heat oil in large skillet over medium-high heat. Add shrimp and garlic; cook and stir 4 to 5 minutes until shrimp are pink and opaque.

2 Add lemon juice, salt, paprika and pepper; cook and stir 1 minute. Remove from heat; discard garlic. Sprinkle with parsley.

Makes 6 to 8 servings

. . . .

Basil-Lime Scallops

SHRIMP AND TOMATO STIR-FRY

20 kalamata olives, pitted and coarsely chopped
1 cup cherry tomatoes, halved
¼ cup chopped fresh basil
¼ teaspoon plus ⅛ teaspoon salt, divided
¼ teaspoon black pepper
2 tablespoons olive oil, divided
1 pound medium raw shrimp, peeled and deveined (with tails on)
1 clove garlic, minced
⅛ teaspoon red pepper flakes
1 medium zucchini, quartered lengthwise and cut crosswise into 2-inch pieces
1 medium onion, cut into 8 wedges

1 Combine olives, tomatoes, basil, ⅛ teaspoon salt and pepper in medium bowl; toss gently.

2 Heat 1 tablespoon oil in large skillet over medium heat. Add shrimp, garlic and red pepper flakes; cook and stir 3 minutes or until shrimp are pink and opaque. Remove to plate.

3 Heat remaining 1 tablespoon oil in same skillet over medium-high heat. Add zucchini, onion and remaining ¼ teaspoon salt; cook and stir 5 minutes or until edges of vegetables begin to brown.

4 Add tomato mixture and shrimp to skillet; cook and stir 1 minute or until heated through.

Makes 4 servings

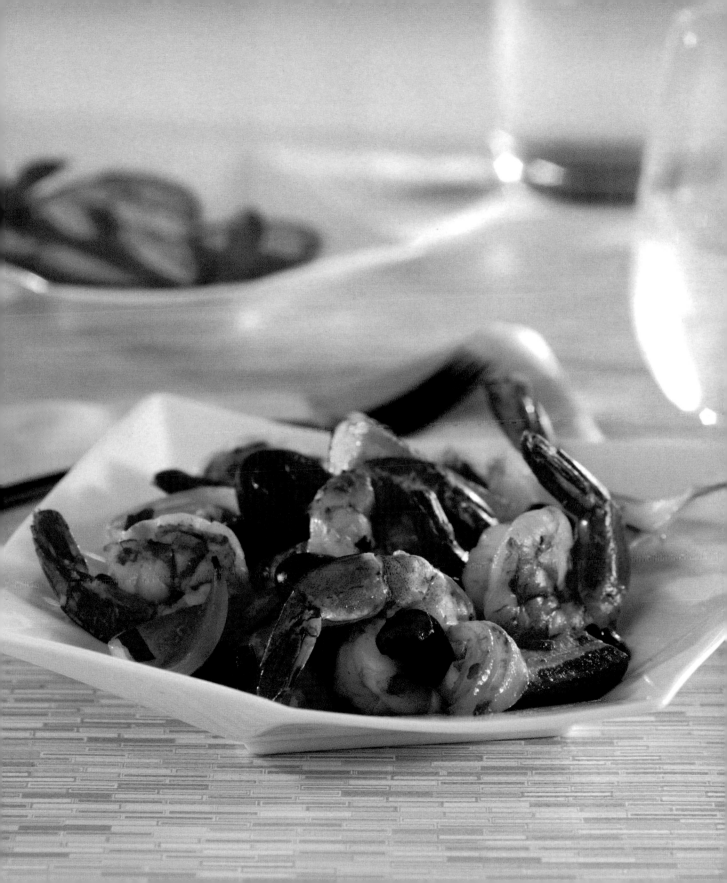

SAVORY SEAFOOD SOUP

- 2½ cups water
- 1½ cups dry white wine
- 1 onion, chopped
- ½ red bell pepper, chopped
- ½ green bell pepper, chopped
- 1 clove garlic, minced
- 8 ounces halibut, cut into 1-inch pieces
- 8 ounces sea scallops, cut into halves
- 1 teaspoon dried thyme
- Juice of ½ lime
- Dash hot pepper sauce
- Salt and black pepper

1 Combine water, wine, onion, bell peppers and garlic in large saucepan; bring to a boil over high heat. Reduce heat to medium-low; cover and simmer 15 minutes or until bell peppers are tender, stirring occasionally.

2 Add halibut, scallops and thyme to saucepan; cook 2 minutes or until fish and scallops are opaque. Stir in lime juice and hot pepper sauce. Season with salt and black pepper.

Makes 4 servings

TIP: If halibut is not available, cod, ocean perch or haddock can be substituted.

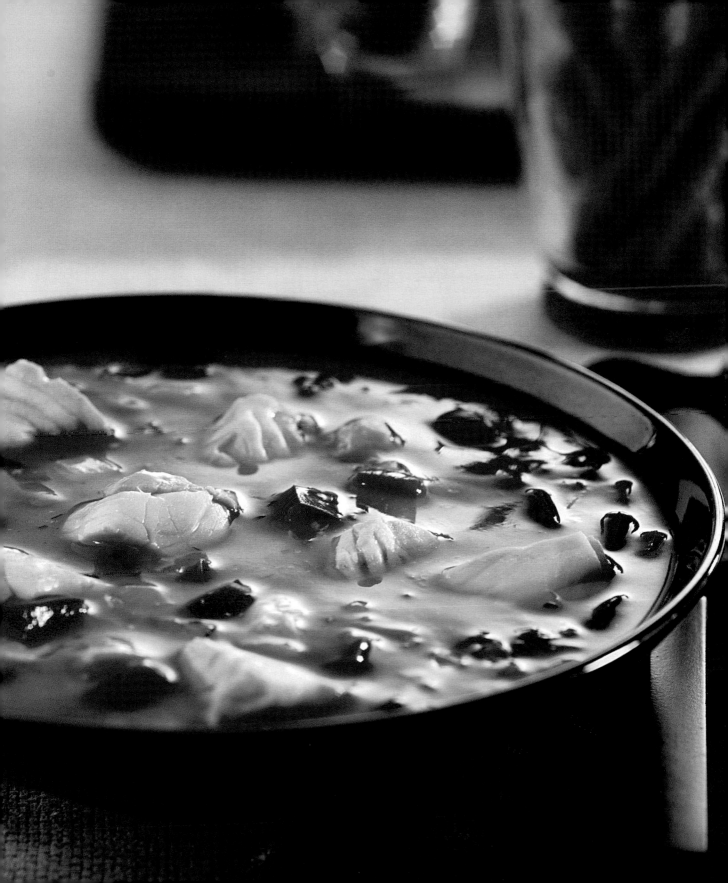

COCONUT SHRIMP WITH PEAR CHUTNEY

Pear Chutney (recipe follows)
½ **cup shredded unsweetened coconut**
¾ **teaspoon curry powder**
½ **teaspoon salt**
3 **tablespoons coconut oil, melted**
1 **pound large raw shrimp, peeled and deveined (with tails on)**

1 Prepare Pear Chutney; set aside. Preheat oven to 425°F. Line baking sheet with foil or brush with oil.

2 Combine coconut, curry powder and salt in shallow dish; mix well. Toss shrimp and coconut oil in large bowl. Coat shrimp with coconut mixture, pressing lightly to adhere. Place on prepared baking sheet.

3 Bake 4 minutes. Turn and bake 2 minutes or until shrimp are pink and opaque. Serve with Pear Chutney.

Makes 4 servings

PEAR CHUTNEY

1 **tablespoon coconut oil**
1 **jalapeño pepper, seeded and minced**
1 **small shallot, minced**
1 **teaspoon grated fresh ginger**
1 **medium unpeeled ripe pear, cut into ½-inch pieces**
1 **to 2 tablespoons water**
2 **teaspoons cider vinegar**
⅛ **teaspoon salt**
1 **tablespoon chopped green onion**

1 Heat oil in medium saucepan over low heat. Add jalapeño, shallot and ginger; cook and stir 3 minutes or until shallot is tender.

2 Stir in pear, 1 tablespoon water, vinegar and salt; cover and cook over low heat 15 minutes or until pear is tender, adding additional 1 tablespoon water if mixture becomes dry. Add green onion; cook and stir 1 minute. Cool before serving.

Makes 2 cups

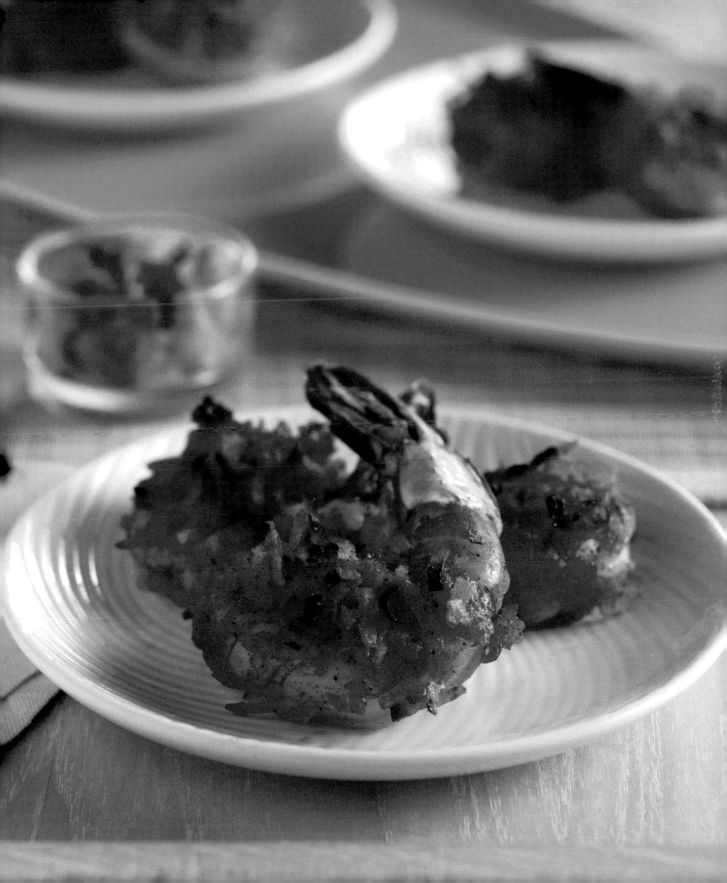

LEMON ROSEMARY SHRIMP AND VEGETABLE SOUVLAKI

- 3 tablespoons extra virgin olive oil, divided
- 2 tablespoons lemon juice
- 2 teaspoons grated lemon peel
- 2 medium cloves garlic, minced
- ½ teaspoon salt
- ½ teaspoon finely chopped fresh rosemary leaves
- ⅛ teaspoon red pepper flakes
- 8 ounces raw shrimp, peeled and deveined (with tails on)
- 1 medium zucchini, halved lengthwise and cut into ½-inch slices
- ½ medium red bell pepper, cut into 1-inch pieces
- 8 green onions, trimmed and cut into 3-inch pieces

1 Oil grid. Prepare grill for direct cooking.

2 Combine 2 tablespoons oil, lemon juice, lemon peel, garlic, salt, rosemary and red pepper flakes in small bowl; mix well.

3 Alternately thread shrimp, zucchini, bell pepper and green onions onto four 12-inch metal or bamboo skewers. Brush with remaining 1 tablespoon oil.

4 Grill kabobs over high heat 2 minutes per side or until shrimp are pink and opaque. Remove to serving platter; drizzle with sauce.

Makes 4 kabobs

NOTE: "Souvlaki" is the Greek word for shish kebab. Souvlaki traditionally consists of fish or meat that has been seasoned in a mixture of oil, lemon juice, and seasonings. Many souvlaki recipes also include chunks of vegetables such as bell pepper and onion.

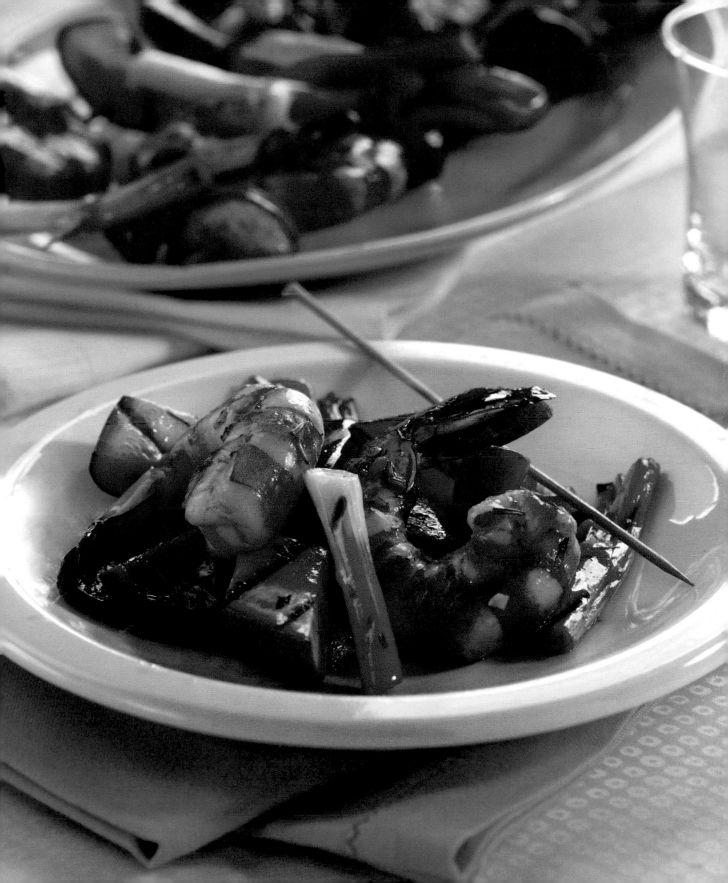

SHRIMP GAZPACHO

1 tablespoon olive oil

8 ounces medium raw shrimp, peeled and deveined, tails removed

½ teaspoon salt, divided

⅛ teaspoon black pepper

3 plum tomatoes, chopped (about 1½ cups)

¼ small red onion, chopped

¼ cucumber, peeled and chopped

¼ cup finely chopped roasted bell peppers, divided

1 clove garlic, chopped

¾ cup tomato juice

1 tablespoon red wine vinegar

1 Heat oil in medium nonstick skillet over high heat. Season shrimp with ¼ teaspoon salt and black pepper. Add to skillet; cook 3 minutes or until shrimp are pink and opaque, turning once. Remove to plate.

2 Combine tomatoes, onion, cucumber, half of roasted peppers, garlic and remaining ¼ teaspoon salt in food processor; process until combined. Add tomato juice and vinegar; process until smooth.

3 Divide tomato mixture among bowls; top with shrimp and remaining roasted peppers.

Makes 2 servings

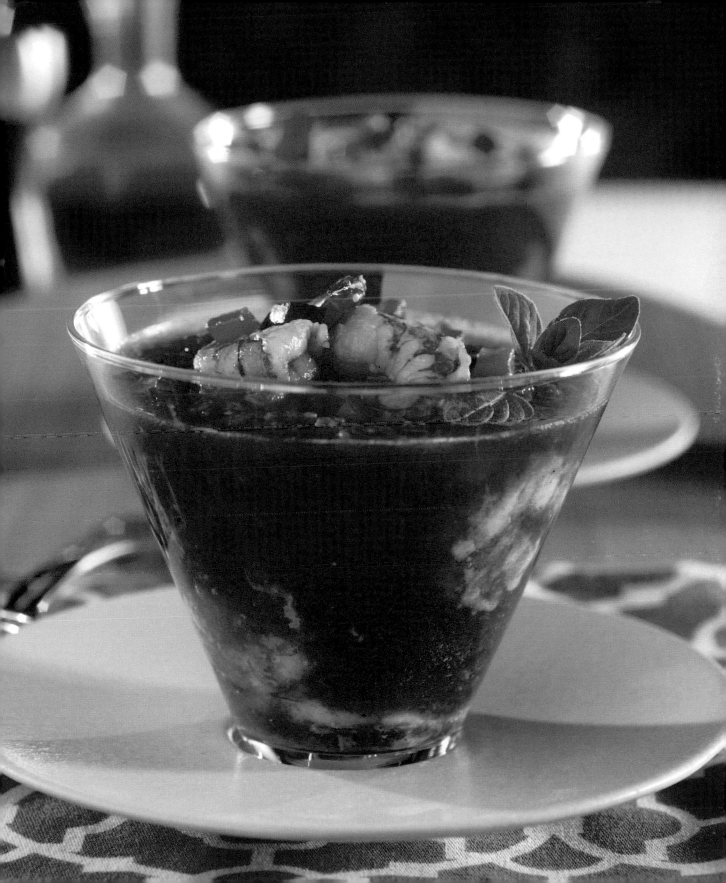

CHIPOTLE SHRIMP AND SQUASH RIBBONS

2 cloves garlic
1 canned chipotle pepper in adobo sauce, plus 1 teaspoon sauce
2 tablespoons water
¼ teaspoon salt
2 medium zucchini
2 medium yellow squash
1 tablespoon olive oil
1 small onion, diced
1 medium red bell pepper, cut into strips
½ pound medium raw shrimp
   Lime wedges (optional)

1 Combine garlic, chipotle pepper with adobo sauce, water and salt in food processor; process until smooth.

2 Shave zucchini and yellow squash into ribbons with vegetable peeler.

3 Heat oil in large skillet over high heat. Add onion and bell pepper; cook and stir 1 minute. Add shrimp and chipotle mixture; cook and stir 2 minutes. Add squash; cook and stir 1 to 2 minutes or until shrimp are pink and opaque and squash are slightly wilted. Serve with lime wedges, if desired.

Makes 4 servings

NOTE: Chipotle peppers are smoked jalapeños. They are usually found canned in adobo sauce, which is a dark red sauce made of chili peppers, herbs, and vinegar. Leftover chipotle peppers in adobo sauce can be frozen in resealable freezer food storage bags or in an airtight container.

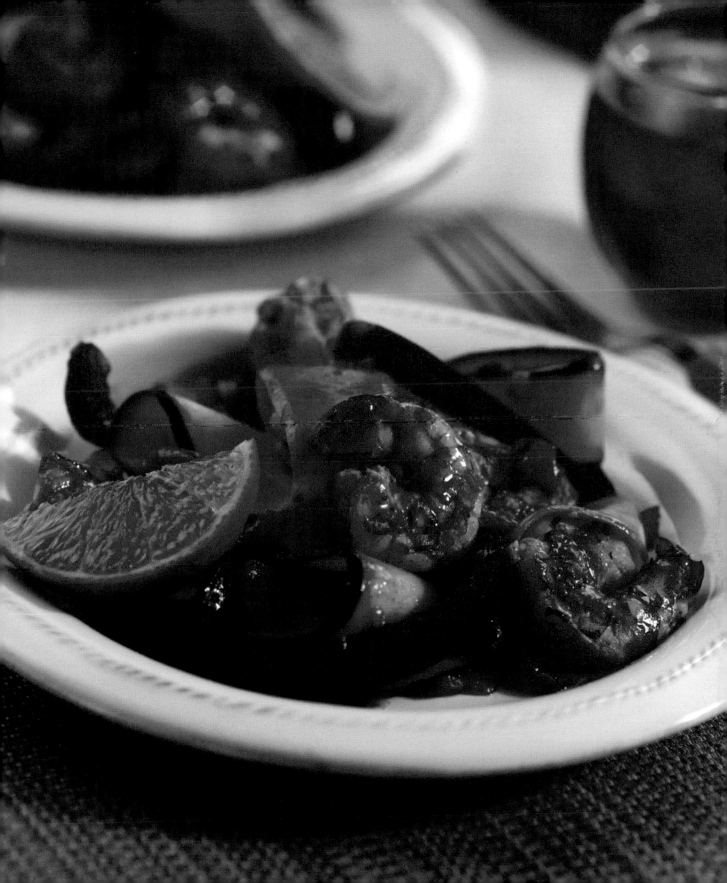

SIDES & SNACKS

ROASTED PARSNIPS, CARROTS AND RED ONION

- 2 carrots, quartered lengthwise and cut into 2-inch pieces
- 2 parsnips, quartered lengthwise and cut into 2-inch pieces
- ¾ cup vertically sliced red onion (¼-inch slices)
- 2 tablespoons extra virgin olive oil
- 1 tablespoon balsamic vinegar
- ½ teaspoon salt
- ⅛ teaspoon black pepper

1 Preheat oven to 425°F.

2 Combine carrots, parsnips, onion, oil, vinegar, salt and pepper in large bowl; mix well. Spread in single layer on jell roll pan.

3 Bake 25 minutes or until tender, stirring occasionally.

Makes 4 servings

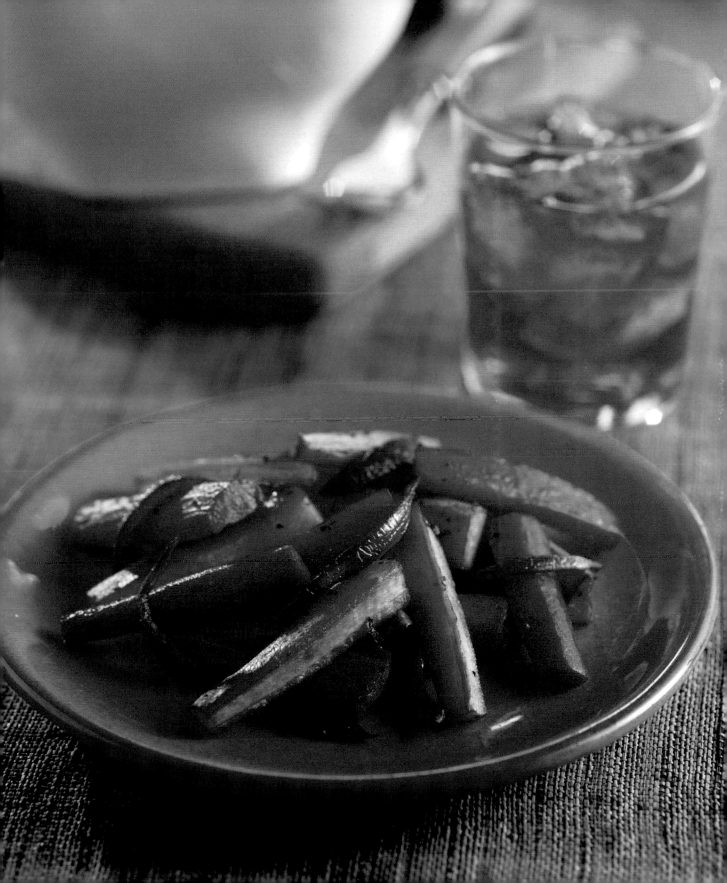

LIME-GINGER COLE SLAW

   2 cups shredded green cabbage
1½ cups matchstick-size carrots
   1 cup shredded red cabbage
  ¼ cup finely chopped green onions
   3 tablespoons lime juice
   2 tablespoons olive oil
   2 tablespoons chopped fresh cilantro
1½ teaspoons grated fresh ginger
  ½ teaspoon salt
  ⅛ teaspoon red pepper flakes

Combine all ingredients in large bowl; mix well. Let stand 10 minutes before serving.

Makes 4 servings

MIDDLE EASTERN SPINACH SALAD

  ¼ cup lemon juice
   2 tablespoons olive oil
  ½ teaspoon salt
  ½ teaspoon curry powder
   1 pound fresh spinach, stemmed and torn
  ¼ cup golden raisins
  ¼ cup minced red onion
  ¼ cup thinly sliced red onion

1 Combine lemon juice, oil, salt and curry powder in small bowl; mix well.

2 Combine spinach, raisins, minced onion and onion slices in large bowl. Add dressing; toss gently to coat.

Makes 4 servings

Lime-Ginger Cole Slaw

SAVORY PUMPKIN HUMMUS

1 can (15 ounces) solid-pack pumpkin
3 tablespoons chopped fresh parsley, plus additional for garnish
3 tablespoons tahini
3 tablespoons fresh lemon juice
2 cloves garlic
1 teaspoon ground cumin
½ teaspoon salt
⅛ teaspoon black pepper
⅛ teaspoon ground red pepper, plus additional for garnish

Combine pumpkin, 3 tablespoons parsley, tahini, lemon juice, garlic, cumin, salt, black pepper and ⅛ teaspoon red pepper in food processor or blender; process until smooth. Cover and refrigerate at least 2 hours. Sprinkle with additional red pepper, if desired. Garnish with additional parsley.

Makes 1½ cups

MARINATED TOMATO SALAD

2 cups cherry tomatoes, cut into halves
1 large cucumber, cut in half lengthwise and sliced
1 large yellow or red bell pepper, cut into strips
3 slices red onion, quartered
2 tablespoons olive oil
2 tablespoons balsamic vinegar
½ teaspoon dried basil
¼ teaspoon onion salt
¼ teaspoon garlic powder
¼ teaspoon dried oregano

1 Combine tomatoes, cucumber, bell pepper and onion in large bowl.

2 Combine oil, vinegar, basil, onion salt, garlic powder and oregano in small bowl; mix well Pour over vegetables; toss to coat. Serve immediately or cover and refrigerate up to 2 hours.

Makes 6 to 8 servings

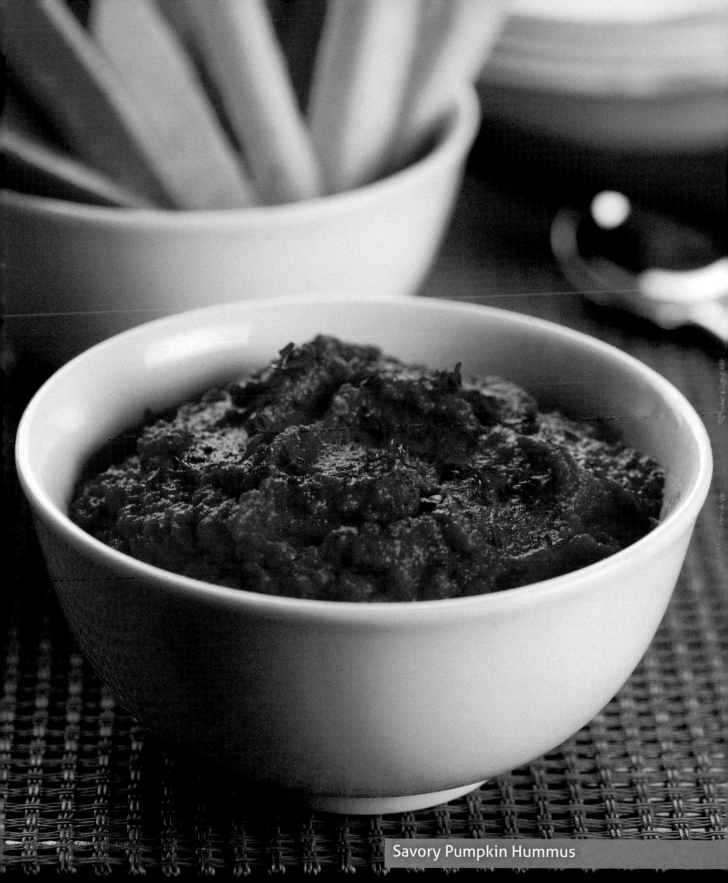

Savory Pumpkin Hummus

SPICY RATATOUILLE WITH SPAGHETTI SQUASH

- 1 spaghetti squash (2 pounds)
- 2 tablespoons olive oil
- 1 small onion, finely chopped
- 1 clove garlic, minced
- 1 small eggplant, diced
- 1 small zucchini, diced
- 1 cup coarsely chopped mushrooms, preferably oyster or shiitake
- 1 can (about 14 ounces) diced tomatoes
- 1 tablespoon minced canned chipotle pepper
- ½ teaspoon salt
- ½ teaspoon dried oregano
- ¼ teaspoon black pepper

1 Pierce squash skin several times with fork or paring knife; place on microwavable plate. Loosely cover with plastic wrap; microwave on HIGH 12 to 13 minutes, turning squash after 6 minutes. (Squash is fully cooked when fork can pierce skin and flesh easily.) Cover and let stand 5 minutes.

2 When squash is cool enough to handle, cut in half lengthwise. Scoop out and discard seeds. Use fork to scoop out cooked squash against the grain and separate into strands. Measure 2 cups squash; cover and keep warm. Save empty squash shells for serving, if desired.

3 Meanwhile, heat oil in large skillet over medium-high heat. Add onion and garlic; cook and stir 1 minute. Add eggplant, zucchini and mushrooms; cook and stir 8 minutes or until vegetables are lightly browned. Add tomatoes, chipotle pepper, salt, oregano and black pepper; cook over medium heat 3 to 5 minutes or until sauce is slightly thickened and heated through.

4 Place squash in squash shells or serving dish; top with ratatouille. Serve immediately.

Makes 4 servings

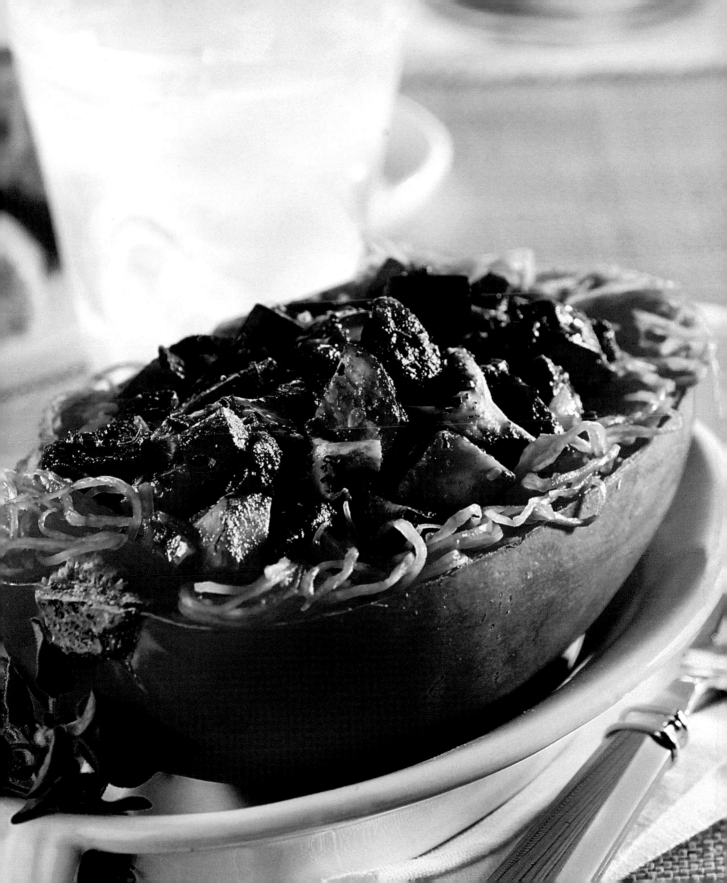

BALSAMIC BUTTERNUT SQUASH

- 3 tablespoons olive oil
- 2 tablespoons thinly sliced fresh sage (about 6 large leaves), divided
- 1 medium butternut squash, peeled and cut into 1-inch pieces (4 to 5 cups)
- ½ red onion, cut in half and cut into ¼-inch slices
- 1 teaspoon salt, divided
- 2½ tablespoons balsamic vinegar
- ¼ teaspoon black pepper

1 Heat oil in large cast iron skillet over medium-high heat. Add 1 tablespoon sage; cook and stir 3 minutes. Add butternut squash, onion and ½ teaspoon salt; cook 6 minutes, stirring occasionally. (Squash should fit into crowded single layer in skillet.) Reduce heat to medium; cook 15 minutes without stirring.

2 Stir in vinegar, remaining ½ teaspoon salt and pepper; cook 10 minutes or until squash is tender, stirring occasionally. Stir in remaining 1 tablespoon sage; cook 1 minute.

Makes 4 servings

GRILLED SESAME ASPARAGUS

- 1 pound asparagus (about 20 spears), trimmed
- 2 teaspoons olive oil
- 1 teaspoon dark sesame oil
- 1 tablespoon sesame seeds
- 2 to 3 teaspoons balsamic vinegar
- ¼ teaspoon salt
- ¼ teaspoon pepper

1 Oil grid. Prepare grill for direct cooking.

2 Place asparagus on baking sheet; drizzle with olive and sesame oils. Sprinkle with sesame seeds, rolling to coat.

3 Grill asparagus over medium-high heat 4 to 6 minutes or until beginning to brown, turning once. Transfer to serving dish; sprinkle with vinegar, salt and pepper.

Makes 4 servings

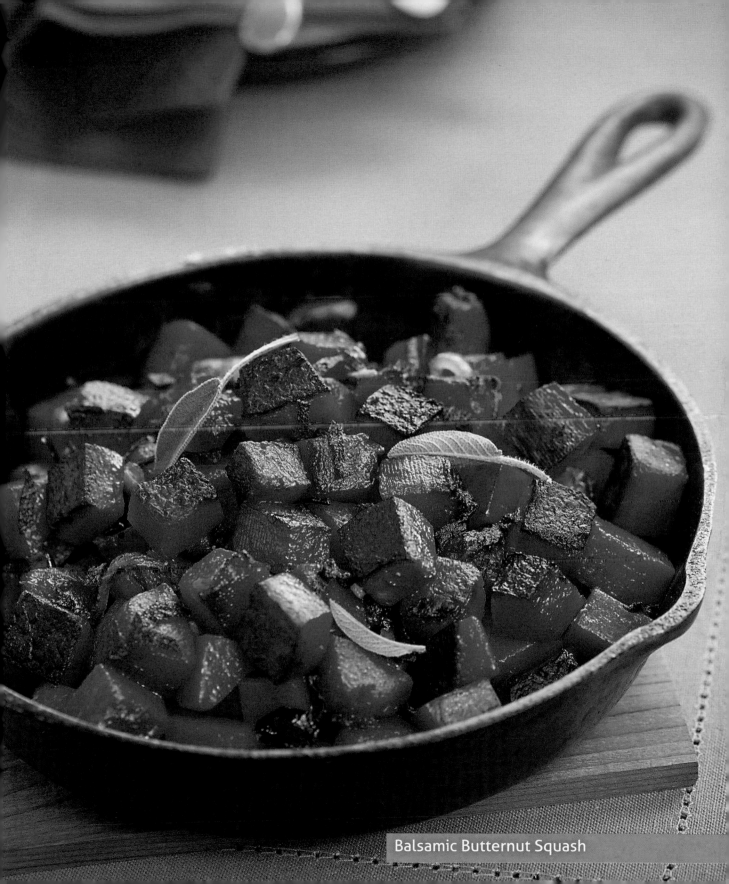

Balsamic Butternut Squash

BEET CHIPS

3 medium beets (red and/or golden), peeled
1½ tablespoons extra virgin olive oil
¼ teaspoon salt
¼ teaspoon black pepper

1 Preheat oven to 300°F.

2 Cut beets into very thin slices, about ¹⁄₁₆ inch thick. Combine beets, oil, salt and pepper in medium bowl; toss gently to coat. Arrange in single layer on baking sheets.

3 Bake 30 to 35 minutes or until darkened and crisp.* Spread on paper towels to cool completely.

Makes 2 servings

*If the beet chips are darkened but not crisp, turn oven off and let stand in oven about 10 minutes or until crisp. Do not keep the oven on as the chips can burn easily.

CRUNCHY JICAMA, RADISH AND MELON SALAD

3 cups thinly sliced jicama
3 cups watermelon cubes
2 cups cantaloupe cubes
1 cup sliced radishes
3 tablespoons chopped fresh cilantro
2 tablespoons olive oil
2 tablespoons lime juice
1 tablespoon orange juice
1 tablespoon cider vinegar
1 tablespoon honey
½ teaspoon salt

1 Combine jicama, watermelon, cantaloupe and radishes in large bowl; mix gently.

2 Whisk cilantro, oil, lime juice, orange juice, vinegar, honey and salt in small bowl until well blended. Add to salad; toss gently to coat. Serve immediately.

Makes 8 servings

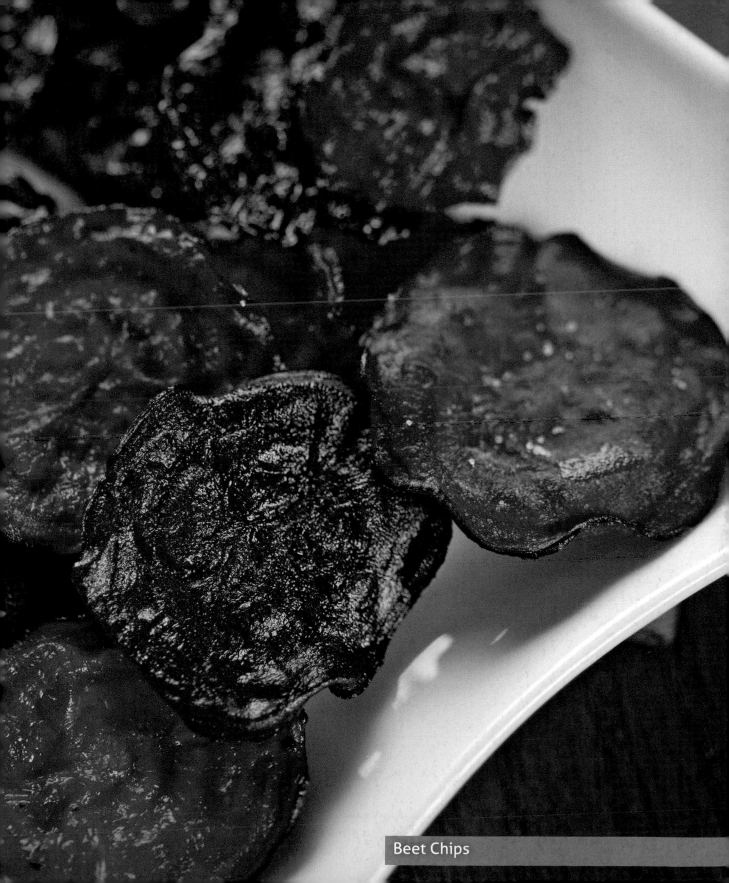

Beet Chips

AVOCADO SALSA

- 1 medium avocado, peeled and diced
- 1 cup chopped onion
- 1 cup chopped peeled seeded cucumber
- 1 Anaheim pepper,* seeded and chopped
- ½ cup chopped fresh tomato
- 2 tablespoons chopped fresh cilantro, plus additional for garnish
- ½ teaspoon salt
- ¼ teaspoon hot pepper sauce

Anaheim peppers can sting and irritate the skin, so wear rubber gloves when handling peppers and do not touch your eyes.

Combine avocado, onion, cucumber, Anaheim pepper, tomato, 2 tablespoons cilantro, salt and hot pepper sauce in medium bowl; mix gently. Cover and refrigerate at least 1 hour before serving. Garnish with additional cilantro.

Makes about 4 cups

MASHED SWEET POTATOES AND PARSNIPS

- 2 large sweet potatoes (about 1¼ pounds), peeled and cut into 1-inch pieces
- 2 medium parsnips (about 8 ounces), peeled and cut into ½-inch slices
- ¼ cup coconut milk
- 1 tablespoon butter
- ½ teaspoon salt
- ⅛ teaspoon ground nutmeg
- ¼ cup chopped fresh chives or green onions

1 Combine sweet potatoes and parsnips in large saucepan. Cover with cold water; bring to a boil over high heat. Reduce heat to low; simmer, uncovered, 15 minutes or until vegetables are tender.

2 Drain vegetables; return to pan. Add coconut milk, butter, salt and nutmeg; mash with potato masher over low heat until almost smooth. Stir in chives.

Makes 6 servings

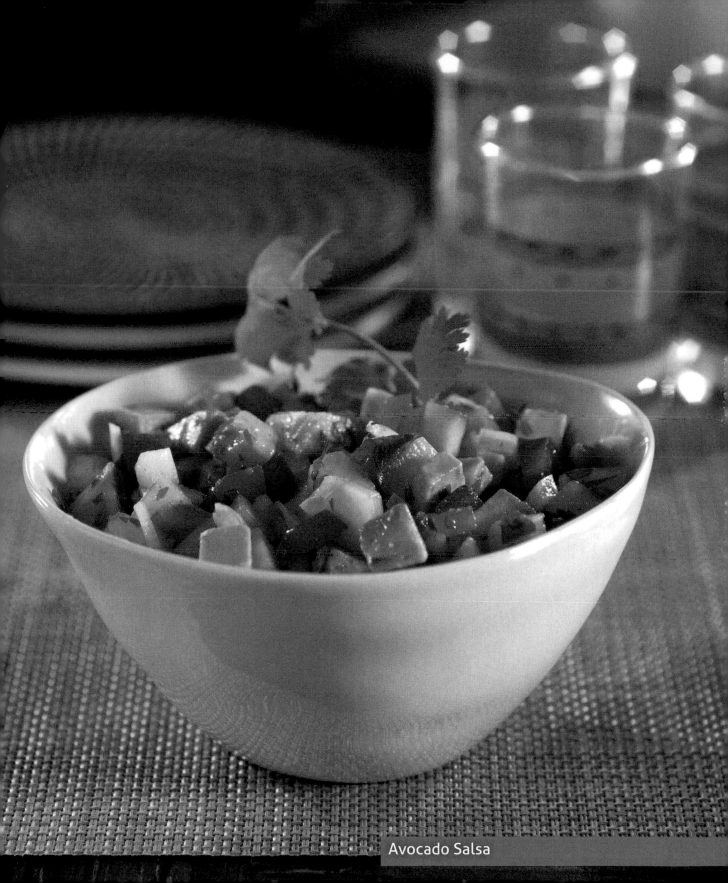

Avocado Salsa

TANGY RED CABBAGE WITH APPLES AND BACON

- 8 slices thick-cut bacon
- 1 large onion, sliced
- ½ small head red cabbage (1 pound), thinly sliced
- 1 Granny Smith apple, peeled and sliced
- 2 tablespoons cider vinegar
- ½ teaspoon salt
- ¼ teaspoon black pepper

1 Cook bacon in large skillet over medium-high heat 6 to 8 minutes or until crisp, turning occasionally. Drain on paper towel-lined plate. Coarsely chop bacon.

2 Drain all but 2 tablespoons drippings from skillet. Add onion; cook and stir over medium-high heat 2 to 3 minutes or until onion begins to soften. Add cabbage; cook and stir 4 to 5 minutes or until cabbage wilts. Add apple; cook 3 minutes or until crisp-tender. Stir in vinegar; cook 1 minute or until absorbed.

3 Stir in bacon, salt and pepper; cook 1 minute or until heated through. Serve hot or at room temperature.

Makes 4 servings

GLAZED MAPLE ACORN SQUASH

- 1 large acorn or golden acorn squash
- ¼ cup water
- 2 tablespoons maple syrup
- 1 tablespoon butter, melted
- ¼ teaspoon ground cinnamon

1 Preheat oven to 375°F. Cut stem and blossom ends from squash. Cut squash crosswise into four slices; scrape out and discard seeds. Place water in 13×9-inch baking dish. Arrange squash in dish; cover with foil. Bake 30 minutes or until tender.

2 Combine maple syrup, butter and cinnamon in small bowl; mix well. Uncover squash; drain water. Brush squash with syrup mixture, letting excess pool in center of squash. Bake 10 minutes or until syrup mixture is bubbly.

Makes 4 servings

Tangy Red Cabbage with Apples and Bacon

BRAISED LEEKS

· · · · · · · · · · · ·

3 to 4 large leeks (1½ to 2 pounds)
¼ cup (½ stick) butter
¼ teaspoon salt
¼ teaspoon black pepper
¼ cup dry white wine
¼ cup chicken or vegetable broth
3 to 4 sprigs parsley

1 Trim green stem ends of leeks; remove any damaged outer leaves. Slice leeks lengthwise up to, but not through, root ends to hold leeks together. Rinse leeks in cold water, separating layers to remove embedded dirt. Cut leeks crosswise into 3-inch lengths; cut off and discard root ends.

2 Melt butter over medium-high heat in skillet large enough to hold leeks in single layer. Arrange leeks in skillet in crowded layer, keeping pieces together as much as possible. Cook about 8 minutes or until leeks begin to color and soften, turning with tongs once or twice. Sprinkle with salt and pepper.

3 Add wine, broth and parsley; bring to a simmer. Cover and cook over low heat 20 minutes or until leeks are very tender. Remove parsley sprigs before serving.

Makes 4 servings

· · · · · · · · ·

TIP: Leeks often contain a lot of embedded dirt between their layers, so they need to be washed thoroughly. It's easiest to slice up to—but not through—the root ends before slicing or chopping so the leeks hold together while washing them.

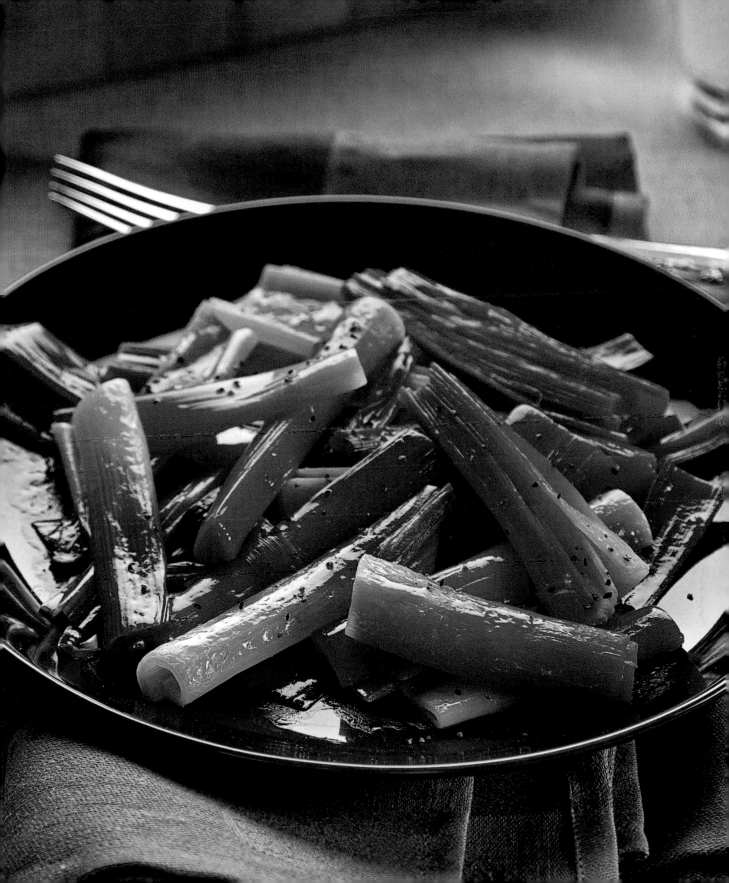

SPINACH MELON SALAD

6 cups packed fresh spinach
4 cups mixed melon balls (cantaloupe, honeydew and/or watermelon)
1 cup zucchini ribbons*
½ cup sliced red bell pepper
¼ cup thinly sliced red onion
¼ cup red wine vinegar
2 tablespoons honey
1 tablespoon olive oil
2 teaspoons lime juice
1 teaspoon *each* dried mint and poppy seeds
½ teaspoon salt

*To make ribbons, shave zucchini lengthwise with vegetable peeler.

1 Combine spinach, melon, zucchini, bell pepper and onion in large bowl.

2 Combine vinegar, honey, oil, lime juice, mint, poppy seeds and salt in small jar with tight-fitting lid; shake well. Pour over salad; toss gently to coat.

Makes 6 servings

BUTTERNUT SQUASH OVEN FRIES

½ teaspoon salt
¼ teaspoon *each* garlic powder and ground red pepper
1 butternut squash (2½ pounds), peeled, seeded and cut into 2-inch thin strips
1½ tablespoons olive oil

1 Preheat oven to 425°F. Combine salt, garlic powder and red pepper in small bowl; mix well.

2 Place squash on large baking sheet. Drizzle with oil and sprinkle with seasoning mix; toss to coat. Arrange squash in single layer.

3 Bake 20 to 25 minutes or until squash just begins to brown, stirring frequently. *Turn oven to broil.* Broil 3 to 5 minutes or until squash is browned and crisp. Spread on paper towels to cool slightly before serving.

Makes 4 servings

Spinach Melon Salad

KALE WITH LEMON AND GARLIC

     2 bunches kale or Swiss chard (1 to 1¼ pounds)
     1 tablespoon olive oil
     3 cloves garlic, minced
     ½ cup chicken or vegetable broth
     ½ teaspoon salt
     ¼ teaspoon black pepper
     1 lemon, cut into wedges

1 Trim tough stems from kale. Stack and thinly slice leaves.

2 Heat oil in large saucepan over medium heat. Add garlic; cook and stir 3 minutes. Add kale and broth; cover and simmer 7 minutes, stirring occasionally. Reduce heat to medium-low; cover and simmer 8 to 10 minutes or until kale is tender.

3 Season with salt and pepper. Squeeze lemon over each serving.

Makes 4 to 6 servings

HERB-ROASTED CAULIFLOWER

     5 cups cauliflower florets
    1½ tablespoons extra virgin olive oil
     ¾ teaspoon dried thyme
     ½ teaspoon salt
     ⅛ teaspoon black pepper
     1 tablespoon finely chopped fresh Italian parsley
     2 teaspoons lemon juice

1 Preheat oven to 425°F.

2 Combine cauliflower, oil, thyme, salt and pepper in large bowl; toss to coat. Spread in single layer on jelly-roll pan.

3 Roast 25 minutes or until tender and brown in spots, stirring occasionally. Transfer to large bowl; stir in parsley and lemon juice.

Makes 4 servings

A

Adriatic-Style Halibut, 130
Apples
 Cinnamon-Spiked Beef and Tomato Stew, 69
 Quick and Easy Pork Chops with Apples, 82
 Spiced Pork Tenderloin and Apples, 102
 Tangy Red Cabbage with Apples and Bacon, 180
Asparagus
 Flank Steak and Roasted Vegetable Salad, 64
 Greek Roast Chicken, 42
 Grilled Sesame Asparagus, 174
 Roasted Dilled Scrod with Asparagus, 140
 Salmon Salad with Basil Vinaigrette, 128
Avocado
 Avocado Salsa, 178
 California Omelet with Avocado, 10
 Grilled Red Snapper with Avocado-Papaya Salsa, 138
 Guacamole, 97
 Pork Tenderloin with Avocado-Tomatillo Salsa, 106
 Southwest Chicken Burgers with Avocado Salad, 45

B

Bacon
 Pork and Cabbage Soup, 80
 Tangy Red Cabbage with Apples and Bacon, 180
Baked Orange Roughy with Vegetables, 144
Balsamic Butternut Squash, 174
Balsamic Chicken, 36
Balsamic Grilled Pork Chops, 78
Basil-Lime Scallops, 152
Basil Vinaigrette, 128
Beef
 Beef and Pepper Kabobs, 72
 Beef Pot Roast, 56
 Beef Tenderloin with High Spice Rub, 48
 Chili á la Mexico, 54
 Cinnamon-Spiked Beef and Tomato Stew, 69
 Cuban-Style Marinated Skirt Steak, 68

Beef *(continued)*
 Flank Steak and Roasted Vegetable Salad, 64
 Flank Steak with Italian Salsa, 70
 London Broil with Marinated Vegetables, 66
 Middle Eastern Beef and Eggplant Stew, 62
 Mustard Crusted Rib Roast, 50
 Rib Eye Steaks with Chili Butter, 58
 Scotch Eggs, 16
 Serbian Lamb Sausage Kabobs, 121
 Skirt Steak with Red Pepper Chimichurri, 74
 Steak al Forno, 76
 Swiss Steak Stew, 76
 Texas Meets N.Y. Strip Steaks, 60
 Warm Steak Salad with Mustard Dressing, 52
Beet Chips, 176
Braised Lamb Shanks with Orange and Rosemary, 110
Braised Leeks, 182
Broiled Cod with Salsa Salad, 126
Broiled Hunan Fish Fillets, 136
Burgers
 Deluxe Mediterranean Lamb Burgers, 120
 Southwest Chicken Burgers with Avocado Salad, 45
 Veggie-Packed Turkey Burgers, 34
Butternut Squash Oven Fries, 184

C

Cabbage
 Lime-Ginger Cole Slaw, 168
 Pork and Cabbage Soup, 80
 Tangy Red Cabbage with Apples and Bacon, 180
 Warm Blackened Tuna Salad, 142
California Omelet with Avocado, 10
Carnitas, 97
Cauliflower
 Herb-Roasted Cauliflower, 186
 Pork Curry over Cauliflower Couscous, 100
Chicken
 Balsamic Chicken, 36
 Chicken Mirabella, 24
 Chunky Chicken Stew, 46

Chicken *(continued)*
Curried Chicken and Winter Vegetable Stew, 40
Ginger-Lime Chicken Thighs, 46
Greek Roast Chicken, 42
Grilled Chicken Adobo, 22
Honey-Roasted Chicken and Butternut Squash, 26
Jalapeño-Lime Chicken, 32
Lemon Chicken, 28
Roast Chicken and Olive Kabobs, 44
Roast Chicken with Peppers, 18
Roasted Rosemary Chicken Legs, 34
Southwest Chicken Burgers with Avocado Salad, 45
Spicy Squash and Chicken Soup, 20
Chili á la Mexico, 54
Chipotle Shrimp and Squash Ribbons, 164
Chunky Chicken Stew, 46
Cider Pork and Onions, 96
Cinnamon-Spiked Beef and Tomato Stew, 69
Coconut Shrimp with Pear Chutney, 158
Crunchy Jicama, Radish and Melon Salad, 176
Cuban Garlic and Lime Pork Chops, 94
Cuban-Style Marinated Skirt Steak, 68
Curried Chicken and Winter Vegetable Stew, 40

D
Deluxe Mediterranean Lamb Burgers, 120
Dilled Salmon in Parchment, 136

E
Easy Halibut Steaks with Tomato and Broccoli Sauce, 146
Egg Dishes
California Omelet with Avocado, 10
Scotch Eggs, 16
Scrambled Egg and Zucchini Pie, 17
Smoked Salmon and Spinach Frittata, 12
Spicy Crabmeat Frittata, 14
Three-Egg Omelet, 17
Eggplant
Middle Eastern Beef and Eggplant Stew, 62
Spicy Ratatouille with Spaghetti Squash, 172

F
Fish
Adriatic-Style Halibut, 130
Baked Orange Roughy with Vegetables, 144
Broiled Cod with Salsa Salad, 126
Broiled Hunan Fish Fillets, 136
Dilled Salmon in Parchment, 136
Easy Halibut Steaks with Tomato and Broccoli Sauce, 146
Greek-Style Salmon, 124
Grilled Red Snapper with Avocado-Papaya Salsa, 138
Grilled Swordfish Sicilian Style, 122
Grouper Scampi, 140
Halibut with Roasted Pepper Sauce, 132
Mustard-Grilled Red Snapper, 130
Roasted Dill Scrod with Asparagus, 140
Salmon Salad with Basil Vinaigrette, 128
Savory Seafood Soup, 156
Smoked Salmon and Spinach Frittata, 12
Spiced Salmon with Pineapple-Ginger Salsa, 148
Tuna Steaks with Pineapple and Tomato Salsa, 134
Warm Blackened Tuna Salad, 142
Flank Steak and Roasted Vegetable Salad, 64
Flank Steak with Italian Salsa, 70
Fresh Plum Salsa, 92

G
Ginger-Lime Chicken Thighs, 46
Glazed Maple Acorn Squash, 180
Greek Leg of Lamb, 112
Greek Roast Chicken, 42
Greek-Style Salmon, 124
Grilled Chicken Adobo, 22
Grilled Red Snapper with Avocado-Papaya Salsa, 138
Grilled Sesame Asparagus, 174
Grilled Swordfish Sicilian Style, 122
Grilling Recipes
Balsamic Grilled Pork Chops, 78
Beef and Pepper Kabobs, 72
Cuban Garlic and Lime Pork Chops, 94
Cuban-Style Marinated Skirt Steak, 68
Deluxe Mediterranean Lamb Burgers, 120
Flank Steak with Italian Salsa, 70

Grilling Recipes *(continued)*
    Ginger-Lime Chicken Thighs, 46
    Greek Leg of Lamb, 112
    Grilled Chicken Adobo, 22
    Grilled Red Snapper with Avocado-Papaya
        Salsa, 138
    Grilled Sesame Asparagus, 174
    Grilled Swordfish Sicilian Style, 122
    Herbed Lamb Chops, 118
    Jalapeño-Lime Chicken, 32
    Lemon Rosemary Shrimp and Vegetable
        Souvlaki, 160
    Moroccan-Style Lamb Chops, 114
    Mustard-Grilled Red Snapper, 130
    Rib Eye Steaks with Chili Butter, 58
    Rosemary-Garlic Lamb Chops, 108
    Serbian Lamb Sausage Kabobs, 121
    Steak al Forno, 76
    Texas Meets N.Y. Strip Steaks, 60
    Veggie-Packed Turkey Burgers, 34
Grouper Scampi, 140
Guacamole, 97

H

Halibut with Roasted Pepper Sauce, 132
Herbed Lamb Chops, 118
Herb-Roasted Cauliflower, 186
Honey-Roasted Chicken and Butternut
    Squash, 26

I

Italian Tomato-Braised Lamb, 114

J

Jalapeño-Lime Chicken, 32
Jerk Turkey Stew, 30

K

Kale
    Chunky Chicken Stew, 46
    Kale with Lemon and Garlic, 186

L

Lamb
    Braised Lamb Shanks with Orange and
        Rosemary, 110
    Deluxe Mediterranean Lamb Burgers, 120

Lamb *(continued)*
    Greek Leg of Lamb, 112
    Herbed Lamb Chops, 118
    Italian Tomato-Braised Lamb, 114
    Moroccan-Style Lamb Chops, 114
    Roasted Dijon Lamb with Herbs and Country
        Vegetables, 116
    Rosemary-Garlic Lamb Chops, 108
    Serbian Lamb Sausage Kabobs, 121
Lemon
    Cuban-Style Marinated Skirt Steak, 68
    Kale with Lemon and Garlic, 186
    Lemon and Garlic Shrimp, 152
    Lemon Chicken, 28
    Lemon Rosemary Shrimp and Vegetable
        Souvlaki, 160
Lime
    Basil-Lime Scallops, 152
    Cuban Garlic and Lime Pork Chops, 94
    Cuban-Style Marinated Skirt Steak, 68
    Ginger-Lime Chicken Thighs, 46
    Grilled Chicken Adobo, 22
    Jalapeño-Lime Chicken, 32
    Lime-Ginger Cole Slaw, 168
London Broil with Marinated Vegetables, 66

M

Maple and Sage Pork Chops, 90
Maple-Mustard Pork Chops, 84
Marinated Tomato Salad, 170
Mashed Sweet Potatoes and Parsnips, 178
Middle Eastern Beef and Eggplant Stew, 62
Middle Eastern Spinach Salad, 168
Moroccan-Style Lamb Chops, 114
Mushrooms
    Baked Orange Roughy with Vegetables,
        144
    Lemon Chicken, 28
    London Broil with Marinated Vegetables,
        66
    Middle Eastern Beef and Eggplant Stew, 62
    Spicy Pork and Vegetable Stew, 88
    Spicy Ratatouille with Spaghetti Squash,
        172
Mustard Crusted Rib Roast, 50
Mustard Dressing, 52
Mustard-Grilled Red Snapper, 130

O

Olives
Adriatic-Style Halibut, 130
Chicken Mirabella, 24
Flank Steak with Italian Salsa, 70
Greek-Style Salmon, 124
Roast Chicken and Olive Kabobs, 44
Shrimp and Tomato Stir-Fry, 154

P

Pear Chutney, 158
Pork
Balsamic Grilled Pork Chops, 78
Carnitas, 97
Cider Pork and Onions, 96
Cuban Garlic and Lime Pork Chops, 94
Maple and Sage Pork Chops, 90
Maple-Mustard Pork Chops, 84
Pork and Cabbage Soup, 80
Pork Chops with Vinegar Peppers, 86
Pork Curry over Cauliflower Couscous, 100
Pork in Chile Sauce, 90
Pork Roast with Dijon Tarragon Glaze, 84
Pork Tenderloin with Avocado-Tomatillo Salsa, 106
Quick and Easy Pork Chops with Apples, 82
Roasted Pork Tenderloin with Fresh Plum Salsa, 92
Sage-Roasted Pork with Rutabaga, 104
Scotch Eggs, 16
Spiced Pork Tenderloin and Apples, 102
Spicy Pork and Vegetable Stew, 88
Zesty Skillet Pork Chops, 98

Q

Quick and Easy Pork Chops with Apples, 82

R

Rib Eye Steaks with Chili Butter, 58
Roast Chicken and Olive Kabobs, 44
Roast Chicken with Peppers, 18
Roasted Dijon Lamb with Herbs and Country Vegetables, 116
Roasted Dill Scrod with Asparagus, 140

Roasted Parsnips, Carrots and Red Onion, 166
Roasted Pepper Sauce, 132
Roasted Pork Tenderloin with Fresh Plum Salsa, 92
Roasted Rosemary Chicken Legs, 34
Rosemary-Garlic Lamb Chops, 108

S

Sage-Roasted Pork with Rutabaga, 104
Salads
Broiled Cod with Salsa Salad, 126
Crunchy Jicama, Radish and Melon Salad, 176
Flank Steak and Roasted Vegetable Salad, 64
Lime-Ginger Cole Slaw, 168
Marinated Tomato Salad, 170
Middle Eastern Spinach Salad, 168
Salmon Salad with Basil Vinaigrette, 128
Southwest Chicken Burgers with Avocado Salad, 45
Spinach Melon Salad, 184
Warm Blackened Tuna Salad, 142
Warm Steak Salad with Mustard Dressing, 52
Salmon Salad with Basil Vinaigrette, 128
Savory Pumpkin Hummus, 170
Savory Seafood Soup, 156
Scotch Eggs, 16
Scrambled Egg and Zucchini Pie, 17
Serbian Lamb Sausage Kabobs, 121
Shellfish (*see also* **Shrimp**)
Basil-Lime Scallops, 152
Savory Seafood Soup, 156
Spicy Crabmeat Frittata, 14
Shrimp
Chipotle Shrimp and Squash Ribbons, 164
Coconut Shrimp with Pear Chutney, 158
Lemon and Garlic Shrimp, 152
Lemon Rosemary Shrimp and Vegetable Souvlaki, 160
Shrimp and Tomato Stir-Fry, 154
Shrimp and Veggie Skillet Toss, 150
Shrimp Gazpacho, 162
Skirt Steak with Red Pepper Chimichurri, 74

Slow Cooker Recipes
    Middle Eastern Beef and Eggplant Stew, 62
    Pork in Chile Sauce, 90
    Pork Roast with Dijon Tarragon Glaze, 84
    Swiss Steak Stew, 76
Smoked Salmon and Spinach Frittata, 12
Soups
    Pork and Cabbage Soup, 80
    Savory Seafood Soup, 156
    Shrimp Gazpacho, 162
    Spicy Squash and Chicken Soup, 20
Southwest Chicken Burgers with Avocado Salad, 45
Spiced Pork Tenderloin and Apples, 102
Spiced Salmon with Pineapple-Ginger Salsa, 148
Spicy Crabmeat Frittata, 14
Spicy Pork and Vegetable Stew, 88
Spicy Ratatouille with Spaghetti Squash, 172
Spicy Squash and Chicken Soup, 20
Spinach
    Middle Eastern Spinach Salad, 168
    Smoked Salmon and Spinach Frittata, 12
    Spinach Melon Salad, 184
Squash
    Balsamic Butternut Squash, 174
    Butternut Squash Oven Fries, 184
    Chipotle Shrimp and Squash Ribbons, 164
    Glazed Maple Acorn Squash, 180
    Honey-Roasted Chicken and Butternut Squash, 26
    Spicy Pork and Vegetable Stew, 88
    Spicy Ratatouille with Spaghetti Squash, 172
    Spicy Squash and Chicken Soup, 20
Steak al Forno, 76
Stews
    Chunky Chicken Stew, 46
    Cinnamon-Spiked Beef and Tomato Stew, 69
    Curried Chicken and Winter Vegetable Stew, 40
    Jerk Turkey Stew, 30
    Middle Eastern Beef and Eggplant Stew, 62
    Spicy Pork and Vegetable Stew, 88
    Swiss Steak Stew, 76

Sweet Potatoes
    Cinnamon-Spiked Beef and Tomato Stew, 69
    Greek Roast Chicken, 42
    Jerk Turkey Stew, 30
    Mashed Sweet Potatoes and Parsnips, 178
Sweet Spiced Tarragon Roast Turkey Breast, 38
Swiss Steak Stew, 76

T
Tangy Red Cabbage with Apples and Bacon, 180
Texas Meets N.Y. Strip Steaks, 60
Three-Egg Omelet, 17
Tuna Steaks with Pineapple and Tomato Salsa, 134
Turkey
    Jerk Turkey Stew, 30
    Sweet Spiced Tarragon Roast Turkey Breast, 38
    Turkey Lettuce Wraps, 25
    Veggie-Packed Turkey Burgers, 34

V
Veggie-Packed Turkey Burgers, 34

W
Warm Blackened Tuna Salad, 142
Warm Steak Salad with Mustard Dressing, 52

Z
Zesty Skillet Pork Chops, 98
Zucchini
    Chipotle Shrimp and Squash Ribbons, 164
    Lemon Rosemary Shrimp and Vegetable Souvlaki, 160
    London Broil with Marinated Vegetables, 66
    Scrambled Egg and Zucchini Pie, 17
    Shrimp and Tomato Stir-Fry, 154
    Shrimp and Veggie Skillet Toss, 150
    Spicy Ratatouille with Spaghetti Squash, 172
    Spinach Melon Salad, 184
    Veggie-Packed Turkey Burgers, 34
    Warm Blackened Tuna Salad, 142

METRIC CONVERSION CHART

VOLUME MEASUREMENTS (dry)

1/8 teaspoon = 0.5 mL
1/4 teaspoon = 1 mL
1/2 teaspoon = 2 mL
3/4 teaspoon = 4 mL
1 teaspoon = 5 mL
1 tablespoon = 15 mL
2 tablespoons = 30 mL
1/4 cup = 60 mL
1/3 cup = 75 mL
1/2 cup = 125 mL
2/3 cup = 150 mL
3/4 cup = 175 mL
1 cup = 250 mL
2 cups = 1 pint = 500 mL
3 cups = 750 mL
4 cups = 1 quart = 1 L

VOLUME MEASUREMENTS (fluid)

1 fluid ounce (2 tablespoons) = 30 mL
4 fluid ounces (1/2 cup) = 125 mL
8 fluid ounces (1 cup) = 250 mL
12 fluid ounces (1 1/2 cups) = 375 mL
16 fluid ounces (2 cups) = 500 mL

WEIGHTS (mass)

1/2 ounce = 15 g
1 ounce = 30 g
3 ounces = 90 g
4 ounces = 120 g
8 ounces = 225 g
10 ounces = 285 g
12 ounces = 360 g
16 ounces = 1 pound = 450 g

DIMENSIONS

1/16 inch = 2 mm
1/8 inch = 3 mm
1/4 inch = 6 mm
1/2 inch = 1.5 cm
3/4 inch = 2 cm
1 inch = 2.5 cm

OVEN TEMPERATURES

250°F = 120°C
275°F = 140°C
300°F = 150°C
325°F = 160°C
350°F = 180°C
375°F = 190°C
400°F = 200°C
425°F = 220°C
450°F = 230°C

BAKING PAN SIZES

Utensil	Size in Inches/Quarts	Metric Volume	Size in Centimeters
Baking or Cake Pan (square or rectangular)	8×8×2	2 L	20×20×5
	9×9×2	2.5 L	23×23×5
	12×8×2	3 L	30×20×5
	13×9×2	3.5 L	33×23×5
Loaf Pan	8×4×3	1.5 L	20×10×7
	9×5×3	2 L	23×13×7
Round Layer Cake Pan	8×1½	1.2 L	20×4
	9×1½	1.5 L	23×4
Pie Plate	8×1¼	750 mL	20×3
	9×1¼	1 L	23×3
Baking Dish or Casserole	1 quart	1 L	—
	1½ quart	1.5 L	—
	2 quart	2 L	—